The Heartbeat of Success

The Heartbeat of Success:
A Med Student's Guide to Med School Admissions

Alexa M. Mieses

Foreword by Drs. Irwin Dannis, MD, and Lynne Holden, MD

Cover Art By Kaitlyn A. Musto

Copyright © 2013 Alexa M. Mieses

All rights reserved.

ISBN-10: 1491261854
ISBN-13: 978-1491261859

DEDICATION

To Suky, my love, friend and biggest supporter.

CONTENTS

	Foreword	ix
1	Introduction	1
2	Who Should Read This Book?	4
3	All Things Academic	6
4	Extracurricular Activities	20
5	Letters of Recommendation	27
6	Research	37
7	Summer Activities	44
8	Personal Statement	49
9	The MCAT	67
10	AMCAS	86
11	Secondary Applications	106
12	Interviews	114
13	Acceptances	136
14	The Summer Before Med School	147
15	Stories For Inspiration	149

Acknowledgements 159

Resource List 160

FOREWORD

The name Alexa Mieses will probably be unfamiliar to you—until now. However she is far from an unknown entity to us since we have known her and been her mentors for six years. It is hard to believe that only one person was responsible for her multiple admirable accomplishments. We are overwhelmed with joy and pride to see the fruition of our mentoring efforts result in producing a true leader who is dedicated to serving the health needs of all!

Alexa was raised by her mother and grandmother in an underserved area of NYC. Free time was limited because of her need to work beginning as a young teenager and continuing through college. Her grades were not perfect but quite impressive; her MCAT score was close to perfect. She graduated from the City College of New York in five years not because she had academic problems but because she just wanted to learn more. In fact, she received several major awards at graduation.

Alexa's free time was devoted to caring for the underserved, especially in Harlem. She has organized several health fairs in Harlem, mentored and inspired countless students, held leadership positions in several organizations, and even done original research at the National Institutes of Health. Medicine has been her dream for a very long time. She has extensively investigated and experienced what medical school requirements really consist of. Is it any wonder that she quickly accumulated acceptances to six prominent medical schools, half of which offered her full or three-quarter scholarships?

She is now a second year medical student in the dual degree MD/MPH program at the Icahn School of Medicine of Mount Sinai and has decided to share her outstanding knowledge about medical school acceptance. Both of us have had extensive experience with medical school admissions-our combined total is over 45 years. The material she has written is accurate, precise, and real. She has uncovered many of the real secrets of medical school admission. It is presented in a very readable and amusing style. If you really want strategies to succeed in the medical school admissions process, Alexa's book is a must read!

Irwin Dannis, MD
Pre-health Advisor, Mentoring in Medicine, Inc.
Albert Einstein Admissions Committee Co-Chair (Retired)
Member of Admissions Committee for 35 years

Lynne Holden, MD
President, Mentoring in Medicine, Inc.
Associate Professor, Clinical Emergency Medicine, Albert Einstein College of Medicine

The Heartbeat of Success

1 INTRODUCTION

Thus far in life the best advice I've received has come from individuals who know a lot about the experience in question but are not experts in the field. How can someone who is not an expert give great advice? Sometimes experts know too much. They are far removed from the experience and speak in very aspirational and vague terms. It's very easy to forget just how difficult an experience may have been once you've overcome it. On the other hand, someone who just recently experienced what you are about to endure cannot only offer advice but can do so in a way that is meaningful to you. It is for this reason that I have written this book.

I am in no way an expert in the field of medicine. I am a second-year medical student. I've only just begun my medical training. Though I am not yet fully prepared to care for patients (for now), I'm more than qualified to advise premedical students about how to get into medical school. In fact, I have been advising younger students about professional development from the time I was an undergraduate. Since graduating from college and beginning medical school I have continued to mentor high school and college students interested in a career in the health professions. I have held formal and informal mentoring positions as well as given talks, designed workshops and written material about everything premed-related. I was also lucky enough to have amazing mentors of my own. I'm eager to pay it forward.

I grew up in New York City in a working-class family. I attended public school throughout my entire life. I'm the first person in my family to pursue a career in medicine. I'm living proof that with passion, perseverance and the right mentorship, anything is possible.

During my medical school application year, I received fifteen interview invitations. I went on eleven interviews and was accepted to six top-tier medical schools, five in New York. One school offered me a full, four-year scholarship, and two more offered me nearly a full scholarship. I have successfully completed one full year of medical school at the Icahn School of Medicine at Mount Sinai, which is ranked 18th out of 149 medical schools by US News and World Report. I am using my success to guide others and help them achieve their goals.

In addition to my passion for mentoring others, it was only a year ago that my premedical journey came to an end and my life as a medical student began. I vividly remember spending my Saturdays studying organic chemistry reactions at the local coffee shop and reviewing practice MCATs with a fine-toothed comb. It was not that long ago that I had to work up the courage to ask for my first recommendation letter or wait in agony for that first medical school acceptance.

This book will cover all aspects of the medical school application process and describe how to put together an outstanding application. The hardest thing about putting together a medical school application is the fact that you cannot do it overnight. You cannot even do it in one year. Your motivation for choosing to become a physician is often born long before you decide to become "premed" or sit down to write the first words of your personal statement. This book deals specifically with aspects of your application that begin with your undergraduate career all the way through beginning medical school.

I will tell you what I tell all my students. Take every bit of advice with a grain of salt. You should consult doctors, teachers, mentors, premed advisors and admissions committee representatives. Try to hear as many perspectives as possible and lay every piece of advice out like cards on a table. Use what you have been told to find a solution that fits your life and your individual situation. There is no single way to do something correctly. This book communicates just one perspective—a student's perspective—and I hope you find it meaningful.

2 WHO SHOULD READ THIS BOOK?

This book is for undergraduate premedical students and high school seniors interested in applying to medical school. This book will be especially useful to students who are the first in their family to pursue medicine or possibly even the first to attend college. However, a lot of what is written here can apply in other instances. Second-career adults embarking on a new journey to medicine can also benefit from what is written here. Additionally, tips about balancing college courses with extracurricular activities, asking for letters of recommendation, writing personal statements and preparing for interviews can be applied to other career goals and job hunts. This book may also be useful for family members and loved ones of soon-to-be physicians. This book can shed light on exactly what it takes to get into medical school.

The chapters are arranged in the order in which you should think about each component of the medical school application process. Additionally, interwoven throughout each chapter I share personal stories and stories and material from real premeds and their applications. All names, places and dates were changed to protect the identity of the students but the stories and application material are real.

3 ALL THINGS ACADEMIC

When I first started college, I had not yet declared a major. I was torn between majoring in psychology, biology or English. I love all three subjects and choosing one felt like such a big commitment. I was also so preoccupied with what I thought medical schools wanted to see, rather than with doing what I loved.

Finally, in my sophomore year, I committed to biology. I wanted to pursue a subject more tangible than psychology and knew I could continue to write and read on my own—I did not have to major in English. I actually ended up completing a minor course of study in psychology and continuing to pursue writing on my own. The added benefit to majoring in biology was that all of the premedical courses were also part of my required coursework for my major; I killed two birds with one stone.

Despite all of the stones I saved up killing those birds, I decided to spend more time in college anyway! I spent an extra year in undergraduate school that allowed me to do a few things I would have been otherwise unable to do: I studied abroad in Madrid, Spain; I took an acting class; I took a history class about women and medicine; I took a poetry class; I took a creative writing class; and I was a very active servant of my community. Most premedical students are so focused on graduating in four years that they don't have time to do anything else.

Overall, I do not have any regrets. I sometimes wish that I would have majored in English since I spend all my time studying science now as a medical student. My decision to spend an extra year in college was untraditional by many standards but I knew that I would enjoy myself more that way. Medical schools were very interested to learn about my decision and pleased to learn about all I had accomplished as a result of this choice.

Choosing a Major

I'm often asked, "Do I have to major in premed to go to medical school?" For starters, at many colleges "premed" is not a major but a track. This means you must take certain courses (usually courses required by medical schools for admission) to complete the premed track but you major in something else. Additionally, medical schools accept applicants who major in anything as long as they earn a bachelor's degree before beginning medical school. This means you can major in whatever you want!

The only rule about choosing a major is make sure it is one you love! You will spend most of your class time in college completing coursework related to your major, so why would you choose something that "looks good" but in which you have only a slight interest? If you love the subject, you will enjoy learning the material and spend time studying. This means that you're more likely to get higher grades. Even more important than good grades is the opportunity for admissions committees to learn about your passion. What better opportunity is there than to describe why you have chosen your major?

I've also met many students who are interested in becoming physicians but major in something like biomedical engineering as a "back-up." This is a big no, no. First, in many ways majors like engineering are more grueling than premedical coursework. Don't give yourself mountains of unnecessary work because you're afraid you may not be accepted to medical school. This can hurt you in the long run. Second, medical schools never want to hear that you're unsure about the path you've chosen. Should you be invited for an interview, stating that you chose your major in order to have a back-up plan is a huge red flag. The admissions committee will question your motivation for applying to medical school.

On the other hand, let's pretend you started out as a biomedical engineering major as a college freshman. During your time as a biomedical engineering major you realized what you really love is science overall and you have a passion for helping people. So you decided to change your major to biology and enter the premed track. That is all perfectly okay by med school admissions standards. In this case, you pursued biomedical engineering for genuine reasons and along the way discovered you want to become a physician. This does not make you seem unreliable. This is an honest tale of discovering what you are truly passionate about. Now if you change your major ten times, we're back in the red flag zone.

Another very important thing to remember is that you do not have to choose a major right away. Many colleges will allow you to choose a major as late as your second year. If this is the case at your college, and you're not exactly sure what you want to major in, that's fine. You should use the first year of college to explore your interests and gain some focus. You can take general education requirements that are required for graduation in any department (for example an English class or social science class like psychology) in addition to introductory level classes in subjects in which you are interested in majoring. You may discover that you really love art history and that you actually dislike psychology.

Once medical school begins it becomes increasingly difficult to make time for things unrelated to medical school. This theme continues throughout medical training. Therefore, another way in which you may want to choose a major is by choosing something completely unrelated to medicine. You can major in dance, history, music, Spanish, visual arts—whatever! College should be seen as an opportunity to explore all you'd like to explore before committing to a lifetime of training and learning as a physician. By opting to major in something unrelated to science, you may actually give yourself more time to study for premed track classes. You will also be able to experience something new and admissions committees may find you more intriguing. However, don't forget my only rule about choosing a major: only choose a major if you love it—not because you think it will "look good" to admissions committees.

Adjusting to Life as a College Student

Many people believe they have to follow the cookie cutter method of getting into medical school: spend four years in undergraduate school and then go straight to medical school. This cannot be any more false. You want to make sure you perform as well in college as possible. If that means that you do not take biology during your freshman year then so be it. If that means that you want to spend five years in college instead of four, then go ahead! Just make sure that whenever you deviate from the traditional premedical journey that you have a good reason for doing so. You will need to explain to medical schools in your application or during interviews why you chose to deviate from the usual method.

I bring this up because it is important that you do well during your first semester of college. Yes, it is true that some medical schools will cut you slack for bad grades in your first year; they may attribute poor grades to the college adjustment period. But imagine if you did not have bad grades at all? Imagine if you appeared to be well-adjusted to college right from the get go? Medical school admissions committees would love to see this!

One way to do this is to ease yourself into the college experience.

College is an exciting time. For many, it is the first time they're away from home, living alone or living on a budget. College is also very different from high school because you are no longer a child. Even though you are still technically a teenager when you begin college, you will be treated like a young adult. Many professors do not have a strict attendance policy and you will be forced to learn to manage your time. You'll have to balance school work with extracurricular activities, social activities, and for some, a job.

Given that there are so many things to juggle, you want to have control over as many factors as possible. To begin, choose your first semester course schedule wisely. By the end of college, you may feel comfortable taking five or six classes per semester but in the beginning start off slowly. Consider taking the minimum number of classes required to be a full-time student (this varies from school to school but is approximately 12-15 credits or 4 classes).

In order to be productive and ensure you do well, choose two general education requirements (classes that are required for graduation regardless of which major you eventually pursue). For example, many colleges require that their students take a certain number of English courses, a certain number of social science courses, a certain number of classes related to art, so on and so forth. Look up these requirements and choose two general education requirement classes. This way, you are not wasting time, and immediately working towards graduating.

The other two classes you choose to take during your first semester should be related to your major. Or if you have not yet chosen a major, the other two classes should be introductory classes for majors you are considering. Some examples are introductory biology, music appreciation, introductory psychology, introduction to communication and media arts. This will allow you to either pursue your major or explore different majors while maintaining a good grip on your time management skills.

During your first semester of college, it would be great if you did not have to hold a job. I know this is not possible for everyone, as I had to work to support myself throughout college. However, if you must work, try to find a student-friendly job.

A student-friendly job is a job in which you have a lot of down time and/or a very flexible supervisor. A student-friendly job can also be one without any downtime but in some way directly serves your career goal. Some examples of student-friendly jobs with a lot of down time are receptionists or security guards. With a lot of down time, you can still study even if you have to work an eight hour shift. Any job with a flexible supervisor is also considered student-friendly as you may need to take off a day from work in order to prepare for final exams or pursue another scholarly activity. Even jobs like tutoring, which don't have any down time, can still be student-friendly. As a tutor you can often make your own schedule, and you are reinforcing knowledge that can be useful to you in your future coursework or on exams. Another example of a job that may not have a lot of down time but can directly serve your career goal is something like a medical office assistant. The bottom line is you want a job that requires a small investment of your time or has a flexible schedule, and yields huge benefits for you and your goals.

Lastly, an entire chapter in this book discusses extracurricular activities. For now, I will discuss extracurricular activities within the context of beginning college. During the first semester attend different student group events. You may also try volunteering with different organizations, enroll in a knitting class or even join an extreme sports interest group. It's okay to bounce around a bit while you figure out what interests you most. You may actually meet new friends by sampling all the activities your school has to offer. Find one group that is devoted to a topic, cause or activity that interests you; make sure you feel comfortable with most of the other members of the group as well. Do you want to join a supportive group or a group that encourages competition among members? Do you want to join a premedical society? Do you want to join a cooking club? Perhaps you want to organize a clothing drive on campus? These are all things to think about. Only you can decide what is best for you.

After the first semester, reflect on your performance. What were your grades like? What was your stress level like? Do you still feel healthy physically and mentally? If you are still happy and healthy, think about whether you feel ready to take on more responsibility. You can take one extra course during your second semester...or not. You can finally take on a part-time job for some extra money...or not. During the second semester you can also commit to one student group or organization. Think about taking on a leadership role in that organization in addition to attending the group's events and meetings. You should aim to take on a leadership role in some capacity by your second year of college. There is no single rule of thumb regarding these matters. You have to be honest with yourself and find a balance between challenging yourself personally and professionally, without overwhelming yourself.

Alphabet Soup: GPA, D's, F's, P's and W's

Students often want to know what the required minimum grade point average (GPA) is to be accepted to medical school. Unfortunately, there is no easy answer. A high GPA sounds great but if you have a low MCAT score or did not participate in any extracurricular activities you may not be accepted. On the other hand, a student with an average GPA but an outstanding MCAT score who was active in her community may be accepted to medical school.

Rather than fixate on a minimum GPA, let's think about your GPA in terms of trends. You may have had a rocky first semester or maybe a less than stellar first year. If you continued to improve your grades each semester, medical schools would look upon this favorably despite low grades in the beginning. On the other hand, medical schools would frown upon an applicant that had very inconsistent grades. Doing very well one semester and then poorly the next and then better and then worse will make it difficult for medical schools to predict your performance as a medical school student. If they cannot predict how you will perform as a medical student, they will not want to accept you to their school. Ideally, you should do well every semester.

Doing well means getting A's and B's (mostly A's) in all of your courses. It's okay to have a few C's every now and then but only if you genuinely had a very difficult time with the material. In other words, earning a C because you had a difficult time in the course is not the end of the world, as long as earning Cs does not become a pattern. If you do not earn mostly A's and B's every semester, then at least aim for an overall upward GPA trend during your time in college.

The other important thing to know about your GPA is that there is a difference between your overall GPA, your science GPA and your major GPA. Your overall GPA is your grade point average for all of the classes you took in college. Your science GPA only counts the math and science courses you have taken (usually, biology, chemistry, math and physics). Your science GPA will include all of the premed track courses as well as other math and science courses you have taken. Your major GPA takes into account only the courses required for your major. If you are a student who majored in science or math of some kind, your science GPA and major GPA may overlap or be exactly the same.

Your college may or may not calculate these different GPAs for you, but regardless the American Medical College Application Service (AMCAS) application will calculate an overall and science GPA for you when you submit your application. Medical schools require this for review of your application.

I'm highlighting the differences between these GPAs because you want to make sure each of them is strong. You want each of these GPAs to be as consistent as possible. You do not want a strong overall GPA and a weak science GPA or vice-versa.

The other matter to consider is that of D's, F's, P's and W's. D's and F's refer to course letter grades while P's refers to "pass" and W refers to "withdrawal." Allow me to explain.

At the end of each course you take in college, you will receive a letter grade. Clearly, you want to avoid F's and D's whenever possible. However, things in life sometimes go wrong. If you earned an F or a D in a course, you must first try to figure out why you earned a poor grade. Did you take on too many extracurricular activities? Did you not study enough? Did you study a lot but still have trouble understanding the material? Did you understand the material but have difficulty memorizing it? Do you need to improve your writing skills? Again, only you can answer these questions.

Once you have figured out what went wrong, you need to devise a strategy to prevent the problem from occurring again. For example, you may want to cut down your hours at your part-time job, get a tutor for the class or visit your school's writing center to improve your skills. Then you should retake the course.

You should retake the course for two reasons. First, you should demonstrate that you can do better. Medical schools will admire your perseverance. Second, for all premed track classes that medical schools require for admission, an F or a D is unacceptable; you have no choice but to retake the course. If you find yourself in a bit of a limbo, earning a low grade in a course but not failing (e.g. C+), do not plan to retake the course. Instead, you can take a course in the same subject but at a higher level—and you better do well! Nothing looks better than performing well in a more difficult course. Of course, you should only plan to take a more difficult course once you've figured out what went wrong the first time around. You definitely do not want to want to earn another bad grade!

Some colleges offer another course option: taking a course "pass/fail." This means that instead of earning a specific letter grade at the end of the course, you still get credit for the course and either pass or fail. Your transcript will read P or F no matter what your actual numerical grade was in the course. You definitely do not want to frequently take courses "pass/fail." More importantly, medical schools do not permit applicants to take premed track courses "pass/fail."

The only time you should consider taking a course pass/fail is if you absolutely, positively believe you cannot do well in a course but need it to graduate. For example, let's say you are an English major who loves comparative literature and absolutely, positively hates writing poetry. Let's say that your college requires all English majors to take at least one poetry class. Then, it may be okay to take the poetry class pass/fail, especially since poetry is not a premed track course.

The other instance in which you may want to take a class pass/fail is if you simply want to try something new and it has no impact on your college major or premed track. For example, let's say you need one last elective class to graduate and you think taking an acting class would be fun. It may be okay to take the acting course pass/fail since it is simply an elective required for graduation. But remember, you cannot make a habit of taking classes pass/fail. Medical schools want to learn about who you are as a student and person, and they cannot do so if all you have is a bunch of P's or F's on your transcript. If you decide to take a class pass/fail, choose wisely.

Finally, we come to the last letter in our alphabet soup: the W, or withdrawal. This should be avoided at all costs—it should be treated as an F. Most colleges give you a grace period at the beginning of each semester. During this grace period you can drop a course or withdraw from a course without penalty. They allow you to do this in case you realized the course was not for you, it conflicted with another course or simply added too much to your workload. If you drop the course during the grace period, it is simply taken off your transcript. No problem.

Should you decide to drop a course late in the semester, after the grace period, you will receive a W. This is a red flag. A W grade forces admissions committees to believe that you withdrew from the course because you would have otherwise failed. It looks like you were trying to cover up a potential F.

However, please keep in mind that things in life sometimes go wrong. Sometimes you will have to withdraw late in the semester if, for example, you come down with appendicitis or experience a family emergency. In this case, it may be better to earn a W rather than an F (as a W usually does not bring down your GPA but an F does). You will have space on your medical school application to explain why you received a W. Therefore, as with F's, D's and P's, you do not want to make a habit of earning W's. Only withdraw from a class as an absolute last resort. Remember, in some cases it is better to earn a C+ and do better in a more difficult course than to just drop the course all together.

4 EXTRACURRICULAR ACTIVITIES

What's all the fuss about extracurricular activities? Isn't doing well in your coursework and on the MCAT enough to get into medical school? Nope. Extracurricular activities and employment are opportunities to explore your interests, become involved in your community, develop a project or earn money to support yourself. Saying you love to help people during a medical school interview is not enough—actions speak louder than words!

In addition to having a job, I participated in a lot of extracurricular activities during college. I loved every single one of them. Despite having a GPA high enough to be part of the premedical honor society on campus, I chose to devote my time to the premedical club that focused mostly on health equity and professional development: the Minority Association of Premedical Students (MAPS), the undergraduate arm of the Student National Medical Association. I was so passionate about the organization's work and it showed; as a result I was chosen to be Secretary and then President of the local chapter.

During my sophomore year of college, I was awarded the Jeannette K. Watson Fellowship. The JK Watson Fellowship is a two year fellowship that provides professional development opportunities for promising undergraduates; the program's main component is three paid summer internships. Around the same time, I was accepted to a very popular premedical summer enrichment program. I felt torn; should I choose the fellowship or the traditional premedical experience? I ultimately chose the JK Watson Fellowship because I felt more excited about the opportunities it offered.

Once again, pursuing my passion led to positive results. As a Watson Fellow I was able to teach children at the Bronx Zoo, publish a magazine article about HIV/AIDS at Gay Men's Health Crisis and travel to South America to work with at-risk youth through a small charity organization in Santiago, Chile. I chose to do what I loved and medical schools clearly saw my passion shine through my application.

What are Extracurricular Activities?

Let's first define extracurricular activities. Extracurricular activities are activities you engage in outside of class and apart from studying. This includes but is not limited to shadowing a physician, volunteering your time for a certain cause, being part of a student group, holding a job or pursuing a hobby.

Not all of your extracurricular activities need to be related to medicine. There are many things you can pursue that will still speak to the fact that you would make a great physician. For example, you can be a leader with your religious organization, teaching religious instruction to children every Saturday. At first, this may seem unrelated to medicine. However, a closer look tells the admissions committee two things. First, it tells the committee a bit about who you are and how you enjoy spending your free time. Second, you are demonstrating that you are a leader who likes working with other people and teaching. These are all qualities of a great physician!

The only rule for choosing extracurricular activities is the same as the rule for choosing a major: make sure you choose activities you love! If you enjoy what you're doing, you're more likely to remain committed to the activity, excel and take on leadership roles. This is what medical schools want to see. They don't want to see an applicant who says they simply attend premedical student group meetings once a month and shadow a physician every now and then.

When choosing extracurricular activities, choose only a few and remain committed to them throughout your undergraduate career. In doing so, you are allowing yourself to get to know your peers, prepare to take on a leadership role and eventually get a letter of recommendation from whomever supervises the group.

A leadership position doesn't just mean that you became the President of a group. Leadership could also mean that you were in charge of a planning or fundraising committee or created a new service project and led the initiative. Leadership can also mean that you did not hold a formal position at all, but improved the way in which your group delivers supplies or services to the community.

Remember, when you are first adjusting to college, it is okay to bounce around different organizations and student groups until you find the ones you enjoy most. You should commit to your extracurricular activities by the end of your first year of college and stick with them!

Aside from choosing a few activities you love, and remaining committed to them over an extended period of time, there is one more guiding principle to choosing extracurricular activities: choose varied experiences. I advise students to find one clinical activity, one activity that serves your college community and one activity that either serves you as an individual or your community at large. By following this practical formula, you are ensuring that medical school admissions committees see different sides of your personality.

It is important to find a clinical experience because without one, medical school admissions committees may think that you have an unrealistic idea of what it means to be a doctor. Look for a formal program for premedical students that incorporates shadowing (see the Resource List), or find a physician or hospital who will take you on as a volunteer and stick with it! It's better to shadow at one location or with one doctor once a week for 2 years, than to shadow random physicians for an hour here and there, for four years. In addition to learning what it is like to be a physician and an opportunity to interact with patients, you may be able to ask the physician you shadow for a recommendation letter.

An easy way to have fun, demonstrate leadership and serve your community is to become active with a student group on campus. This will ensure that you develop relationships with your peers and possibly even a faculty member as most student groups have faculty advisors. You can join a premedical club, cultural society, religious group, or honor society— whatever! Just make sure the group is productive and works to sponsor events for a good cause. A poetry club that sponsors a poetry slam fundraiser or a "big sib/little sib" program to mentor freshman students are great examples. Remember, it does not have to be directly related to medicine. It just as to be something you enjoy and something productive.

The final type of activity to choose is either something completely self-serving or something that serves the larger community (i.e. your city, your state, the nation etc.). The self-serving activity can be anything you want, but again it has to be productive. For example, if you play an instrument you can list this as an activity on your medical school application. In addition to practicing, it would be great if you also participated in a musical performance or wrote a song (even if it's just an open mic session at the local bar). Engaging in hobbies you enjoy is also a great way to stay sane when school becomes stressful, and to maintain a good balance between work and your personal life. Hobbies do not always have to be something grandiose either. Perhaps you enjoy building model cars. That's great! Maybe you can create your own instruction manual to demonstrate leadership in this area.

Do you see where I'm going with this? Through an individual hobby, you can still demonstrate your ability to be a leader and follow through on projects. You can demonstrate your ability to manage your time and challenge yourself. You can still show the admissions committees who you are. You can show the committee that you will be a great doctor.

The other option I mentioned is more community service. I mentioned this because for some people, community service is their hobby and passion. They would rather do more community service than engage in a hobby like drawing or cooking. That is totally okay. I specified choosing an activity that serves a larger community just for the sake of variation. You will have an opportunity to work with people outside of your college. Some examples are volunteering with national organizations like the Red Cross, Boys and Girls Club or Habitat for Humanity.

In summary, make sure you sample different extracurricular activities if you are undecided about what to pursue. Once you know what you like, choose no more than a handful of activities to commit yourself to over a long period of time. Spend time getting to know your peers and supervisors involved with each activity. Take on leadership roles. When the time comes to apply to medical school, you will have a long and strong history of commitment to meaningful activities that tell the committee who you are and why you will be a good physician.

5 LETTERS OF RECOMMENDATION

During my first semester of biology, I did very well. I decided to take the second semester of biology with the same professor. Again, I did very well. I had visited the professor a few times during his office hours. During that same year, I was applying to a fellowship program and asked my professor for a letter of recommendation. This was the first recommendation letter I had ever asked for in college. Everything seemed to have gone smoothly. I was even accepted into the fellowship program.

Years later, I discovered what was written in that letter of recommendation:

To whom it may concern:

Alexa Mieses was a student in my Bio 101 and Bio 102 classes. She had perfect attendance and earned an A in both courses.

Thank you,
Professor X

WHAT A DISASTER! Thankfully, the fellowship staff saw my potential (and thankfully, also required two letters of recommendation and not just one). The following will describe how to avoid a situation similar to my first recommendation letter experience.

What's a Rec Letter and How Do I Get One?

All medical schools require a letter of recommendation, also known as a rec letter, for admission. They often require one from your college's premedical committee or your premedical advisor, and a second letter from someone who has worked with you in a professional capacity (often a professor in a premed course). While two is usually the minimum number of letters to submit, you can submit more than two. Some medical schools set a maximum number of rec letters as well. Make sure you research each school and verify what its requirements are regarding letters of recommendations (more on this in the AMCAS chapter).

The person who writes your rec letter can be called your "recommender." The recommender's letter should state their name, position/title, how he or she knows you and for how long. Then the letter should go on to describe what makes you special and why you would make a great physician. The purpose of a letter of recommendation is for medical schools to be able learn about who you are and from a reliable, professional source. After reading the letter, medical school admissions committees should feel like they learned something new about you that goes beyond your GPA,

MCAT score or what is written elsewhere in your application. After reading the letter, the admissions committees should be thirsty for more!

The most powerful letter will come from a person who has known you for an extended period of time. The person should have worked with you in a professional capacity (friends, family, or neighbors, definitely cannot write you a letter). Finally, the recommender should know you very well—not just your grades but who you are as a person.

That's a tall order. How on earth are you going to find someone who knows you well, for a long period of time and who is not your grandma to write you a letter of recommendation? Premedical students often ask me this. The short answer is that you have to start to create professional relationships and begin to collect letters of recommendation early on during your undergraduate career.

After each course you finish in college, reflect on your performance in the course. Did you earn good grades? Were you present at each session (physically as well as mentally)? Did you have an opportunity to speak with your professor for something other than help with homework or an exam? Did your professor get to know you and learn about your motivations for wanting to become a doctor? If you answered yes to one of these questions, then you may have found yourself a good recommender.

However, it is not that easy. Simply earning good grades and speaking with your professor during office hours is not enough. One semester is usually not a sufficient amount of time to truly get to know someone. Therefore, try to take more than one class with your potential recommender. For example, perhaps you did well in your freshman English class and really liked the professor. Find out whether this professor teaches more advanced coursework, perhaps a literature, poetry or critical reading class and enroll in the course.

When you take a second course with a professor, make sure you perform at the same academic level as before (or better), and continue to make an effort to allow the professor to learn about you. In this way, the professor will have more opportunities to learn about who you are—and not just about the grade you earned in his or her class. At larger colleges where the class size is large, working on an independent project with a mentor is a huge advantage because your mentor can write you a fantastic letter of recommendation (more on this in the Research chapter).

It is very difficult to find a balance between cultivating relationships with professors for a future letter of recommendation and being a stalker. I cannot tell you how many times I've seen students practically harass professors or follow them to their office every day after class to ask silly questions about the course. Do not do this. It can backfire and make you look like a fool or brownnoser rather than a mature, intelligent, premedical student.

To naturally shine, make sure you are doing what you love! If you are taking courses you enjoy, you are more likely to do well and participate in the course. You may naturally even have thoughtful questions and comments to share with the professor. When you are interested in a course, your professors become interested in you. This rule applies to obtaining letters of recommendation from other people as well: volunteer organization supervisors; student group faculty advisors; employers; physicians; research mentors. If you are passionate about something, you are more likely to truly engage in the work and become a leader. Your personality is more likely to come to the surface. You are more likely to be able to ask for and receive a wonderful letter of recommendation.

How to Ask For a Letter of Recommendation

When you are finally ready to ask someone for a letter of recommendation, make sure you are prepared. You can approach the recommender in person or send them an email in order to arrange a separate time to meet. Do not approach a professor or supervisor years after you worked with them and expect them to remember you. Ask for a letter of recommendation whenever your experience with that person is coming to an end (e.g. the class is over, your research project is over or you have found a new job). Make sure you do not put your recommender on the spot or make him feel rushed. You must ask for a letter of recommendation well in advance of any medical school application or program deadline.

Once you have coordinated a time to meet with your recommender, have a copy of your resume, unofficial or official transcript and a draft of your personal statement ready to go. You should also have some information about the program to which you are applying; it should include general information about the school, program or scholarship to which you are applying, instructions on how your recommender should submit the letter and the submission deadline.

Bring all of these documents with you in a folder to the meeting; this packet is called your dossier. Your recommender should already know who you are but you want to make sure they know very well the program to which you are applying, why you are applying and why you should be accepted. You also want to give these documents to your recommender so that he can include specific details about you that he may not remember off the top of his head but are included in your transcript or personal statement.

However, there is one very difficult thing you must do before you hand over these sacred documents. You must ask your recommender if he feels comfortable writing a STRONG rec letter on your behalf! I say this is difficult because it often feels awkward to ask someone whether or not he can write a strong letter of recommendation for you. However, you must, must, must ask this. I cannot emphasize this enough. Do not pressure your recommender into writing a letter. Give the person the opportunity to turn you down if he so wishes.

Believe it or not, many recommenders will tell you outright that they cannot write a good letter for you. If he does not feel he knows you well enough or long enough, doesn't have time to write a letter because he is busy, or simply does not think you are a strong candidate for the program, then you do NOT want him to write you a letter. Kindly say you understand and thank him for his time.

Even a mediocre letter of recommendation can hurt your application. Lukewarm letters of recommendation make admissions committees wonder why the person did not write an outstanding letter for you and often feel it has something to do with you (rather than your recommender's ability to write). Imagine what an outright negative letter of recommendation can do to your chances of admission to medical school!

The other factor that complicates this issue is that you are technically not allowed to see what the recommender writes. Along with your dossier, you should submit a letter with your signature that waives your right to view the letter of recommendation. Almost all medical schools will not accept a letter of recommendation if they know you have read it; if you have access to the letter then there is always the chance that you coerced your recommender or that your recommender is not being completely honest about the way he feels about you.

Despite this, some recommenders will still allow you to see the letter. They may even ask you to write something for them to include in the rec letter. Do not ever ask a recommender to break the rules for you in this way. If he (on his own) decides to share his letter with you, terrific but keep that information to yourself.

Allowing students to view their letters of recommendation even after they have waived their right to do so is an unauthorized but common practice. This is something professors, advisors and admissions committees will not tell you as it is not permitted—yet still this practice goes on. If you are lucky enough to see your letter of recommendation before it is submitted, keep it confidential. To outwardly admit that you have seen the letter is to render it useless and could even call your ethics into question.

Back in the world where everyone follows the rules, you are not allowed to see your letters of recommendation before they are submitted by your recommender. So how do you really know whether or not someone has written you a good letter? You don't. That is why it is so important to do all the pre-work beforehand: make sure your recommender meets the criteria for a good recommender; make sure you have made a good impression on the recommender; make sure you ask the recommender whether he feels he can write a good letter of recommendation for you and that you have provided him with your dossier!

Once the recommender has agreed to write the letter, leave him alone! Let him work! Two weeks before the submission deadline, send him a friendly email to remind him about the deadline and ask whether he needs any more information from you. Normally, recommenders will notify you once they have submitted the letter. If you do not hear from the recommender two days before the submission deadline, it is okay (and appropriate) to email him again or approach him after class to follow up.

Backups

If you are submitting an application for something with a fast approaching deadline (in other words, you asked for a letter of recommendation very late), you should consider having a back-up recommender. If you asked for a letter too late, the first recommender may miss the submission deadline.

A backup recommender is also appropriate if you have not heard from your first recommender at all and the submission deadline is just days away. There is always the small chance that your first recommender will forget all about your letter and leave you hanging out to dry. Of course, this is the absolute worst case scenario. If you did all the pre-work and actually have a good recommender, this should never happen to you. It's just another thing to consider if you are pressed for time.

Storing Letters and Maintaining Confidentiality

Visit your school's premed office and see if they have a system in place to confidentially store letters of recommendation on your behalf. My school had a system like this in place and it is difficult to imagine another effective way to confidentially store recommendation letters. Although we used a paper-based system, many schools now have an electronic system.

In addition to preserving confidentiality, this allows you to save letters from freshman year and submit them for your medical school application in junior or senior year. Your recommenders can write letters of recommendation for medical school (for the AMCAS application) and submit it to the premed office even though you will not actually apply to medical school for a while. This also gives recommenders outside of school (e.g. employers, physicians, supervisors) a place to submit your letter. Finally, most premed offices will "filter" your recommendation letters. While you are not allowed to view your letters, the premedical office can do so; the office cannot tell you what is written in the letter but can tell you whether a letter is good or that you should find another recommender before submitting your application.

6 RESEARCH

When you hear "research" what pops into your mind? Many people imagine scientists wearing white coats, in a laboratory mixing liquids in test tubes. This image is not wrong, but it is certainly not the only type of research that exists. Briefly, research is any type of scholarly project that seeks to answer a question. Research can be scientific (e.g. chemistry, biology, physics, earth science, engineering), social (e.g. psychology, sociology) or clinical (this means the research involves humans or is patient-centered). You can also conduct research in public health and epidemiology, literature, history, almost anything you can imagine! Even evaluating the effectiveness of a program, project or initiative in your neighborhood is considered research. The whole idea behind research is that you are engaging in a scholarly activity outside of class, asking a question and systematically investigating in search of an answer.

I am no stranger to research, specifically biomedical research. As an undergraduate, I completed a neuroscience honors thesis project. I spent two years working in a laboratory at my college, examining eye movements in humans. I was given a scholarship and award for my thesis. After graduation, I spent one year as a full-time research fellow at the National Institutes of Health (NIH). At NIH, I was working on a project that used behavioral and basic science methods to examine drug addiction. During the summer between my first and second year of medical school, I completed a clinical research project at the Seaver Autism Center with support from the American Academy of Child and Adolescent Psychiatry. My project described the behavior and development of children with Phelan-McDermid Syndrome, a genetic syndrome responsible for approximately 1% of all cases of autism. I enjoy research very much and hope to incorporate it into my career. The following information is based on my experience with research thus far.

When Should You Begin?

I do not recommend doing research during your first year of college. Of course, there are people who do it and love it. However, I'm all about easing yourself into new experiences and ensuring you do well. I even caution doing research during your second year of college as you want to ensure you are ready to seriously engage in scholarly work outside of the classroom without compromising your grades. There are some people who never do research in college and that is okay too. Do not feel obligated to do research just because you think that is what med schools want to see. You should only do it if you're curious about the research experience or passionate about the research subject.

From the time you begin college, keep an eye out for subjects that interest you. This goes hand in hand with choosing a major. You may want to do research to delve deeper into a topic with which you're already familiar, complete a thesis project for your major, or learn about something entirely different and unrelated to your major. Once you have a broad sense of what topics interest you, you can begin to identify a project.

Identifying a Project and Finding a Mentor

By now, you might be able to predict what you're about to read: when you are searching for a research project, start by choosing a topic you love! Nothing is worse than working on a project you could not care less about.

Once you have a subject in mind, you need to understand the research environment at your school. Try to figure out whether your school has a particularly strong department that leads the field. This could be any department, not just a scientific one. You should begin by reviewing your school's website to see which faculty members are conducting research.

This needs to be said right away. As an undergraduate, you should never be expected to design your own project from start to finish. Medical students aren't even expected to design their own projects from start to finish. You should always work under someone who has a lot of research and teaching experience. This person is called your project mentor, research mentor, thesis advisor or principal investigator (PI), depending on the circumstances. Let's stick with "mentor" for now.

While you will choose the broad subject you wish to study and then find a mentor, your mentor will normally be the person who designs the project. There is usually room for you to give your input if you don't feel comfortable with something or if you are especially curious about a specific issue. However, your mentor should be the main project designer. He or she may even give you an assignment that builds upon results from a project that has already been completed by another member of the research group.

Your role as an undergraduate will be to familiarize yourself with published literature related to your project. You may have to be trained in order to learn to perform the techniques or methods necessary to carry out your project. You will collect and analyze data. You will then interpret your results and think about ways to build or improve upon what you discovered. Your mentor should be with you, every step of the way, to guide and support you.

Since mentors are absolutely essential for a good research experience, it is imperative that you find a great mentor! Usually, information about faculty and research projects can be found within the faculty member's department. Speak with other students who are further along in their college career to learn about their experiences; they can tell you about which professors may act as great mentors. You can visit the library and ask the librarian to help you search the literature for research papers written by faculty members at your school. You can also set up informational interviews with faculty.

The purpose of an informational interview is to extract information from the person with whom you are meeting. You may want to learn about what type of research projects the faculty member is working on, whether he or she is taking on new undergraduate students to mentor and what his or her philosophy is on mentoring. You also want to get a feel for the faculty member's personality. Is she approachable? Laid back? A micromanager? What is the culture like among other members of the faculty member's research group (if applicable)? Is it collaborative? Are there a lot of undergraduates or mostly graduate students?

Finding the right mentor is about knowing who you are and under which circumstances you work best. Do you need to be in a highly individualized environment in which you are your mentor's only mentee or do you prefer to collaborate with other students? Do you want someone to create a schedule for you or do you prefer to keep your own hours? If you are someone who is a self-starter and enjoys independent work, then a mentor who is very "hands-on" or a micromanager may not be the best for you. You may want a mentor who is regularly available for advice and support but allows you to work mostly independently. However, if you are the type of person who works best under strict deadlines or you are conducting your first research project, you should have a mentor who is a bit stricter.

To be perfectly honest, the project mentor is more important than the specific project topic. It is better to have a great mentor than to have found the perfect research topic. A terrific mentor will challenge you but make you feel supported, can determine whether or not you complete your project, can determine whether you will have a publication, poster or presentation based on the project, and can write you a wonderful letter of recommendation, as previously mentioned.

Results

Icing on the research cake is having a tangible product result from your work. A tangible product can include a thesis paper (a detailed description of your project from start to finish, usually submitted to your school). Another tangible product is a poster or oral presentation summarizing your work, often presented at local or national conferences devoted to your subject of research.

Sometimes an undergraduate can publish a paper in a peer-reviewed journal based on his or her project; the undergraduate will write the paper and be listed as the first author. This is very rare as often undergraduates do not possess the foundation of knowledge nor technical skill to independently see a project through from inception to publication. However, it does sometimes happen. More common (yet still relatively rare), an undergraduate student may be listed as an author on a publication someone else in the group is writing, but not as the first author. This depends on how much the undergraduate (you) is involved with the other person's project.

At the end of the day, the thing that matters most is that you have found a project you enjoyed or a mentor with whom you enjoyed working. While tangible products really are icing on the cake, the one tangible product for which you can realistically aim is a letter of recommendation. A letter from a mentor who knows you well and for an extended period of time, and has seen you work, will go a long way during the medical school application process.

7 SUMMER ACTIVITIES

By the time you finish your first year of college (or any year of college), you may be exhausted and ready to do nothing but relax. Not so fast. If you are serious about becoming a physician, then you should use your summers in a productive way; there are almost limitless options from which you can choose.

You may choose to take a class to get ahead or try something new. You can either take classes related to your major course of study or an elective required for graduation. It is not recommended that you take premed courses over the summer. There are some instances in which this is okay, but overall medical schools believe that summer courses are easier. As always, you will hear stories about people who took organic chemistry or physics over the summer and still got into medical school.

However, admissions committees want to see that you can juggle difficult courses (i.e. premed courses) during the academic year. This demonstrates your sustained ability to juggle various things and manage your time—a quality absolutely essential to succeeding in medical school.

Another way to spend your summer is by completing a study abroad program. You are not allowed to take premed courses abroad; most medical schools will not count foreign credits for premed track classes required for admission. However, you can take electives or other classes related to your major that do not fall under the premed track. Also, because medical schools will not accept foreign credits for premed courses it is often difficult for premedical students to spend an entire semester or year studying abroad. Don't fret. Short-term study abroad programs are often offered during the summer and allow you to get the study abroad experience without compromising your medical school application. During my first summer of college I spent one month in Madrid, Spain taking Spanish language and Spanish art history courses.

If you are engaged in a research project, the summer is a fantastic way to move your project along. In many cases, colleges will provide undergraduate students with funding to complete summer research. If this is not available at your college, you can also consider applying to summer research programs at other schools and institutions. Institutions across the country have many fellowships and scholarships available for students to complete a research project over the summer. Some programs will even pay for your travel or housing. See the Resource List for more details.

Completing any other type of formalized summer program can also be productive. For example, as an undergraduate I was awarded a professional development fellowship (which I previously mentioned). For two years, the fellowship required us to participate in various activities but the major component was summer internships. For three consecutive summers, I was paid to complete meaningful work through an internship. The internships were not directly related to medicine. I spent my first summer teaching children at the zoo, my second summer in the public policy department of an HIV non-profit organization and my final summer in South America teaching children with special needs. These experiences allowed me to further cultivate and demonstrate my leadership skills as well as serve others. Medical schools truly admired this.

Many people also have to spend their summers working full-time to support themselves. That is totally acceptable. Medical schools will understand if you needed to work and therefore could not participate in some other activity. However, even if you are working full-time, it is important to engage in something that will help your application to medical school shine. Even if you only volunteer in a clinical or non-clinical setting for just an hour a week, make sure you are doing something to highlight your altruism and desire to become a physician.

But How Do I Find These Opportunities?

You must start to plan your summer early on. You cannot wait for the semester to end and expect to find a job, research position, volunteer experience or fellowship. Deadlines for certain programs can be as early as the winter preceding the summer. Even if you wish to study abroad or take a class at your college, registration begins way before the summer does.

It may sound crazy, but start to think about your upcoming summer when school first begins in the fall. By keeping your summer in the back of your mind, you are preparing yourself to take advantage of opportunities that present themselves and to submit an application right away (if necessary). This will also ensure that you have time to ask for letters of recommendation for a given summer program and that you will not miss any deadlines. If you wish to take a class, this will ensure you get the summer class and schedule you want.

You also do not want to wait around for opportunities to fall into your lap. While things sometimes do fall into your lap unexpectedly, you must still be proactive. You must actively seek out opportunities for the summer. A great place to begin your search is at your college. Once you have a broad idea of what you want to do, visit the career center, appropriate department or your advisor for more information about such programs. You can also use a search engine to search the internet for opportunities. You can type in phrases like "premed summer program" or "summer undergraduate research fellowship."

Generate a list of programs you like. You can start a spreadsheet or handwritten list and include the name of the program, what you liked about it, application requirements and deadline. Even if the deadline is very far away (or the application for the upcoming summer has yet to open) keep the program on your list. This will ensure that you are ready to go when the program finally begins to accept applications. For a list of some popular programs, see the Resource List.

Don't be afraid to apply to more than one program. Apply to as many as you are interested in and can manage. Should you be accepted to more than one program, fellowship etc., you can always turn down one program. While it is wonderful to be offered an opportunity, you are free to turn it down if you like. Remember my story about being accepted simultaneously to two summer programs as a sophomore in college. It's better to have too many options than no options at all.

All of this applies for jobs as well. Some employers start to hire in the winter or spring even though you will not officially begin your job until the summer. Many students who wait until the summer to search for a summer job will have a very difficult time finding one. Just make sure that once you commit to something, you stick with it. It is not okay to formally commit to a job (or any other opportunity) and then drop it when something better comes along.

8 THE PERSONAL STATEMENT

The chapters in this book are arranged in the order in which you should be thinking about these topics. Why then, is the chapter about your personal statement before chapters on the MCAT and AMCAS? This chapter is placed here because you need to begin to think about your personal statement early in your career.

Inception

Although your essay may be revised a million more times, it is never too early to begin writing it. You can even begin during your first year of college if you wish to do so. In fact, beginning to write your personal statement does not begin with writing at all. It begins with thinking.

Before you put your pen to paper (or begin typing, for those in the 21st century) you should set aside time for self-reflection. Among the million and one other things you have to do, self-reflection may not sound important. However, I cannot stress enough the importance of this process. In order to write a unique essay that will make a lasting impression on admissions committees you must be self-aware and learn to articulate what you think and feel.

Self-reflection does not have to be a long, drawn out process that takes up your weekend. Even just ten minutes a day can make all the difference. Consider keeping a journal (on paper or on your computer). As you push through your undergraduate years, complete coursework, volunteer, work, conduct research, organize a walk-a-thon—whatever it is—write about it afterwards. There are even dictation software programs that work with a microphone to type what you say. Was there a person you met who inspired you? Was this your first time interacting with a patient? Did you learn something new? What did you enjoy about working with that physician? Writing down small thoughts like these may help you later as you write your personal statement.

In addition to keeping track of the moments, sights, sounds and people you experience in college, you should also reflect on your past. I do not doubt you want to become a doctor to help people, yet your essay must have more substance than that. What events, places or people influenced your decision to become a physician? Why is it so important that you become a physician and not another type of healthcare professional? What does "physician" mean to you?

Finally, think about your future. What do you think life will be like as a medical student? What about as a physician? If you have no idea, start speaking to more medical students and physicians. Organize informational interviews and keep track of these experiences in your journal. Gain clinical experience through shadowing physicians or volunteering in a clinical setting. You don't have to know which specialty of medicine you want to pursue. It's actually better if you keep an open mind. However, you can still think about what will make you a successful medical student and what you hope to achieve as a physician.

Another helpful thing to do in preparation for writing your personal statement is to read others' personal statements. Some examples are included in this book. There are many other books as well specifically devoted to writing a personal statement and include samples. See the Resource List for more information. Browse through sample essays to get an idea of what a personal statement should sound and look like. Notice the length, tone, use of active voice, sentence length etc.

Just Dive In

At some point, you will have to just start writing. If you apply to any special fellowships, scholarships or programs during your undergraduate career, most will require a personal statement as part of the application. This is a great way to begin writing your actual personal statement for medical school. Treat every application you complete as an undergraduate as practice for the real thing (AMCAS).

The Opener

The first paragraph of your personal statement will set the tone for the rest of the essay and (to be honest) your application. You want to command the reader's interest but you have to do so in a way that is professional and sincere. A wishy-washy, boring first paragraph will make your reader want to simply stop reading. However, the personal statement is not an exercise in creative writing. You want to find the perfect balance between grabbing the reader's attention without sounding like a lunatic.

Write concisely. You want the reader to feel as though they can hear your voice. Don't use big words you would not normally use in everyday life, and don't use big words just for the sake of using big words. Also, even though you want the reader to imagine your voice, you cannot write in an informal manner. Remember, this is your medical school application personal statement, not Cosmopolitan magazine. In some cases, the first sentence alone can have a tremendous impact on the rest of your essay.

All of the names, places, dates and other identifying information have been changed in the following excerpts from real personal statements. These personal statements were provided by a very reliable source who worked in medical school admissions for over twenty years. Here are some examples of how NOT to begin your personal statement, from REAL essays that were submitted to medical schools:

> *Since high school, I've been successful at almost everything I do. I'm an excellent athlete, I excel in basketball and football. I fence and swim and have trained for a triathlon. I have a master's degree from a top university and I speak French. I have worked in finance and other business fields as well as jobs related to medicine. I have had one goal in mind, and that is to become a doctor.*

This first paragraph is not only boring and a recitation of accomplishments but makes the applicant sound like a braggart. Everything that he said is unrelated to the last sentence about his goal to become a physician.

> *My name is JJ and I'm 22 years old. I am currently a senior at X University where I have a scholastic scholarship.*

This is neither powerful nor captivating.

> *I couldn't decide what the hell to write about, so I hopped on my motorcycle and took a ride.*

Bad, bad, bad.

> *I spend much time thinking about discoveries in molecular biology which I have made. Certain discoveries of mine either invalidate or supersede basic science concepts mentioned in the 1959, 1968 and 1978 Nobel Awards (8 medals).*

The choice of words and sentence structure is awkward (more on this later). I did not include the rest of the paragraph because the first two sentences are enough. This is a terrible way to start to an essay.

> *Circumcision is a surgical removal of the penis' foreskin. You see, smegma can accumulate under the foreskin, and this formation may eventually result in irritation and infection.*

I'm pretty sure you can figure this one out.

> *Imagine if you will, being away from family and friends. Imagine sitting in a room, engrossed in one's studies. Suddenly, you feel you are no longer alone. You sense a presence, although there are no footsteps or breathing. No words are spoken yet you know something is present. I knew I had to act quickly. I turned to come face to face with that presence in my room. In my wildest moments I had never imagined anything so big, with quite so many appendages. It was a millipede.*

This person was clearly trying to catch the reader's attention. This might not have been so bad if the first paragraph was the start of a story related to discovering she wanted to be a doctor or something scholarly. Instead, the writer continued to write about the millipede for the rest of her ENTIRE essay. This is what I meant about sounding like a lunatic. Additionally, in some places the applicants word choice or sentence structure sound awkward, for example, "In my wildest moments I had never imagined..." I think she meant to say "in my wildest dreams."

> *Turbid ocean churning false perception of hope and fear. Where is he? Have you seen him? My friend of heart and mind, where are you? A sick sensation vibrates through my being. A policeman collects your belongings and I believe the rumor. There is a diver in the chamber. Trembling cracks the beliefs in my mind as it struggles to picture you in the chamber being healed. The words from the dive master "he's dead" open the floodgates and harshly solder my mind and body together. A peaceful experience for you deep in mother ocean's embrace, a spiritual meditation while chaos is rippling at the surface. The mind and heart united in awareness is the source of wisdom.*

I had to read this paragraph a few times before I actually understood what the writer was trying to convey. It should never be that difficult to understand your essay. Additionally, the writer was trying to be descriptive and paint a picture but did so in a way that was ineffective. There are a lot of unnecessary, complicated words. The writer sacrificed meaning in an effort to sound poetic. This not only defeated the purpose of the paragraph, but probably made the admissions committee member not want to continue reading. Don't just write something to get the reader's attention. Instead, discuss a meaningful experience in a way that is easy to understand, honest and sincere—not contrived.

> *I possess an exceptional physique. I'm 6'3" tall and weigh 205 pounds. I have a well-defined and muscular frame. My build is not solely the result of genetics. It is the result of several years of weightlifting and proper body maintenance.*

This person had good intentions. He used his entire essay to compare the discipline and dedication necessary for weightlifting to that required to become a doctor. This was a nice attempt, but overall, a weak analogy. It could have had a much more powerful impact if he made a few minor adjustments, and had a different opening paragraph. This paragraph seems a bit too unconventional and self-promoting.

> *Take a very patient, forty-three year old follicle and introduce an equally aged swimmer. Not Michael Phelps, but a tailed champion butterflier on the microscopic level. Let their merger brew in an amniotic cocktail for nine months, and what do you get? Probably something that slithered out of Hecate's cauldron or myself!*

After a few reads, I realized that this person was speaking about a sperm fertilizing an egg—the author's conception. No one wants to read about that in an essay, especially not in the way this applicant wrote about it. To make matters worse, the paragraph jumped all over the place mentioning a professional swimmer, an amniotic cocktail and Hecate's cauldron. It was confusing and weak opener.

THE HEARTBEAT OF SUCCESS

Do you know how a laser works? Simply stated, it stimulates the emission of radiation by adding energy. When this radiation is released, it adds, in phase, to the energy that was inputted. Think about what that means for a second. Just try to visualize the intensity of the energy, a power of force so concentrated that it can physically burn through matter. Picture now that you have this type of concentrated power flowing through you. Close your eyes for a moment and try to imagine the feeling of total peace, the kind of serenity that lets your mind and soul and body blend together as one. You are no longer in a physical state. You are like that laser, a creation of energy. This is my goal in life.

This applicant went a little too far in trying to "talk" to the reader and it comes off as awkward and borderline unprofessional. Additionally, this paragraph is very long with no indication that it is leading to a meaningful essay. That in itself can have a negative impact on your overall application, despite a potentially meaningful essay.

I am a failure. No, don't try to convince me otherwise; I know I am. While that hopefully served its purpose as an attention-grabber, it is also true. I would not have written it otherwise. What I've come to realize, however, is that failure is by definition but a mere obstacle necessary for success, at least as defined by the Edward Rudner Dictionary. I'll get back to this concept. First let me bore the reader with the story of my life.

This is a good example of everything you should not do in a personal statement. He wrote a radical first sentence just to shock the reader. The way in which he referenced the dictionary seemed off the cuff and awkward. He literally spoke to the reader and even demonstrated poor self-esteem or poor judgment as a writer by referring to his life as boring.

The Body and Conclusion

Even if you have a strong, coherent, captivating opener, the body of your essay has to be just as strong. A personal statement is not a resume. All personal statements have a maximum word limit. Do not waste your precious word allowance by reiterating your entire curriculum vitae. You should only describe an extracurricular activity, class, job, project, or summer experience if it adds something to your story.

When I was in elementary school, my teacher always emphasized one important rule about writing: show don't tell. For certain types of writing, especially for personal statements, it is more effective to show the reader something through your words rather than to simply state it. For example, instead of writing "I'm a hard worker," write about a situation that shows you are hardworking. If you do this properly, you will never have to explicitly say you are hard-working.

When you are completely stumped, you can try this exercise I often tell my students to do. Make a list of 5-10 attributes you think every good physician should have. Then think about examples from your own life in which you demonstrated these attributes. For example, if you say physicians have to love the learning process, you can describe the ways in which you've academically challenged yourself. If you say good physicians are compassionate, you can describe a time in which you interacted with someone (perhaps a patient) and demonstrated compassion.

You should not use exactly what you wrote during the exercise for your personal statement. The purpose of the exercise is to get you to think about what it means to be a physician. Also, it will help you "show" the reader that you would make a good physician rather than just tell the reader. The exercise will give you the starting material to build a great essay.

Many people advise students to have a theme for their essay. This is good advice but it is more important to send the right message than to have a theme. Don't focus on creating a theme. In fact, if you do enough self-reflection and choose the right things to write about in your personal statement, a theme will naturally emerge. In your essay you should define what it means to be a physician (not literally, just use your words to show what it means), why you want to become a physician, what influenced your decision to pursue medicine and what type of impact you want to have on others.

I'll tell you a bit about my essay. Rather than show you my actual essay, it will be more helpful to discuss its structure. I began thinking about my life from start to finish. What inspired my desire to become a physician and how did this interest evolve over time? I also wanted to talk about the "big picture"; what was medicine going to allow me to do in the world?

I started my personal statement with a short paragraph, a vignette, which described my frequent trips to the doctor with my mother (a diabetic). These trips first gave me the idea to pursue medicine. Yet my interest in medicine evolved over time. No child can honestly know what it means to be a physician.

On these trips to the doctor, I saw a lot of fast food restaurants in my neighborhood (more so than in other neighborhoods). At the time, I did not know that this was contributing to the very problems many of my family members and neighbors visited the doctor to resolve: obesity and diabetes. I was witnessing health disparities and did not yet know it. More on this later.

My essay then went on to describe my passion for science. This passion lead me to the Bronx High School of Science, a specialized, competitive, public school for the sciences. However, while a student at Bronx Science several of my classmates died of drug overdoses. This personally had a negative impact on me as I struggled with the idea of my classmates dying so senselessly. These events had a positive influence on my professional life as they sparked my interest in neuroscience and medicine. I saw medicine as a way to combat addiction, mental illness and other health problems. I also started a drug awareness club at school and learned how fulfilling it is to serve others. My desire to become a physician was solidified.

I pursued my passions for medicine and service at my undergraduate institution. My essay described why I chose my major and discussed my volunteer and clinical experiences (e.g. President of a premedical club, organizing a health fair, four years working with a plastic surgeon, four years tutoring underserved children, four years tutoring biology for college students, employment, the professional development fellowship etc.). I discussed these experiences because they were in some way related to my story. In college, I finally learned what the term "health disparities" meant and learned to articulate my interest in public health. I began to see a role for doctors beyond the examination room and in the community as agents of change.

My high school experiences were fresh in my mind as an undergraduate, and I wanted to pursue neuroscience research as a means to learn more about the brain. I completed an honors thesis project in vision science. While my research project was related to neuroscience, it was not related to drug addiction (the initial thing that got me interested in the brain). So I decided to take a year off, apply for and was awarded a full-time research fellowship with the National Institutes of Health-National Institute on Drug Abuse.

I concluded my essay by focusing on the big picture. As a physician I will be able to pursue my passion for service, science and lifelong learning. I will also be able to have a positive impact on society. I believe that mentoring the next generation of physicians (you) is part of my duty. As a physician I hope to resolve health disparities and work with underserved minority populations in an effort to provide them quality healthcare. This big picture idea ties into the vignette I told at the beginning. Voila! Everything I said was for real—except for the "voila" part. If only it were that easy. The truth is I am very proud of my personal statement. However, I spent years writing it.

While you write, do not worry about word length. You can worry about this later. It's easier to write too much and have to cut some things out rather than not write enough. Don't worry too much about spelling yet either. Just focus on telling your story and getting your message heard.

Another situation in which students may find themselves is feeling as though they don't have a story. "I don't know why, I've just always wanted to be a doctor." I often hear this. Even if you did not experience a tremendous life-altering event, I bet you still have a story. Even if you just describe in your essays all the ways in which you help people, you can write an effective essay. Perhaps an encouraging science teacher inspired you to pursue medicine. Self-reflection combined with the exercise I described earlier can help you discover your story.

Revisions

During the year in which you will apply to medical school, it's time to make some serious and final revisions to your essay. The best way to do this is to choose three people to be your essay readers. Beware of having too many people read your essay as numerous comments and revisions can pull you in a million directions. Before you know it, the essay may not sound like yours.

The first person you choose to be a reader is someone who knows you very well, perhaps a family member or friend. This person can read your essay and tell you whether you sound like you or not. A second person should be a mentor of some sort who also knows what is required to be accepted to medical school. This person can be your premedical advisor, a professor, supervisor, research mentor or physician as they should strike a balance between helping you keep your essay unique but also ensure you send the right message to admissions committees. The final person can be an English professor or someone else who is a very proficient writer but may not be involved with medicine. This person's responsibility will be to examine the mechanics of your essay.

A Word about Mechanics

While the content of your essay is paramount, the technical skill you use to write your essay is critical. Any error in writing mechanics can absolutely break your application. It makes admissions committees think you are careless or did not spend time on your essay—this applies to your entire application.

I'm talking about spelling, grammar, punctuation and syntax (word-choice). Make sure you stay within the maximum word or character limit of the essay. There cannot be even one typo. Sometimes word processing programs will not pick up problems related to grammar. For example, make sure you don't confuse "their" with "there" or "they're," "then" with "than," or "compliment with "complement" (like I once did). If you spell these words correctly, word processing programs may not detect that you are using them within the wrong context.

Use sentences of varying length (some long, some short). Get rid of run-on sentences. This will make your essay easier to read. Also, it is often helpful to use the active voice. This is a personal statement. Make it feel personal. It's okay to speak in the first-person or use the word "I." Finally, be yourself. Do not use SAT words because you think it will make you sound smarter. For example, for some reason, students like to use the word "utilize" instead of "use." In most cases, "use" is just fine and "utilize" is actually wrong. Don't look up a synonym for one word. Just say what you mean. Don't overcomplicate things.

Here are some more REAL examples of essays that seriously violate rules of the English language or at least use superfluous language:

> *Last year two weeks before Christmas, I received words from my mother that my student loan for the school year had been repudiated. The realization of withdrawing from college for the Spring semester floored me. I was confused and devastated with my dream of attending medical school seemingly jeopardized. Needless to say I sat through the final examinations without much recollection. The frantic search during Winter break for new loans and scholarships ended in disillusionment. As a result, it was an extremely depressed Christmas. But I decided to fight on even though it appeared to be an impossible mission.*

This applicant chose the wrong words to describe the challenge he faced. For example, "depressed Christmas" makes it sound as though the holiday itself was depressed. The applicant should have written, "It was a very depressing Christmas" or "I was extremely depressed during Christmas." Furthermore, the applicant should have simply reworded the entire sentence and said something like "there wasn't any cheer that Christmas." There are also problems with punctuation (the "s" in "spring" does not need to be capitalized).

One day I stumbled upon Stephen Covey's The Seven Habits of Highly Effective People. While reading the book and contemplating Covey's central dogma of the paradigm shift, it became brilliantly self-evident the source of any inspiration must be the manifestation of internal virtue. In my search for an external source of gratification I had lost sight of the ascendancy of personal power. My initial propensity to ascribe to football the dictation of my character presumed an inseparability between exterior and interior principles. I had mistaken proto-cooperation for dynamic necessity, the channel for the foundation. While the loss of external medium did compromise the synergism, it did not preclude the existence or materialization of my innate ideals.

Whoa. Enough said.

I have a big purpose for my life, that is self-development. I would like to challenge something every time, and those challenges can led development of myself. One reason why I am studying at University X is that I wanted to place myself in the severe situations since universities back home are very easy to keep up and to graduate. Since I had language problems when I entered my college, taking higher courses are very hard job. There are some factors to motivate me to do something...When I study something or learn how to do, I always try to have some interests in it.

There is no doubt this applicant did not speak English as a first language. That is totally okay! I'm not trying to poke fun at the applicant for having trouble with English. What I would like to point out is that this essay could have been radically improved if only the applicant asked for help. If this applicant found three people to help with revisions, this could have been an entirely different and effective essay.

9 THE MCAT

For many, this is the first chapter you will read. You may have skipped everything and jumped right to this page in an effort to learn about the dreaded MCAT. *Dun dun dun*! For others, this may be the first thing you ever read about the MCAT. Many premedical students become fixated on the MCAT. Please allow me to start off with the following: the MCAT is not a measure of your intelligence—it's just a measure of how well you take that specific exam. Many studies have shown that standardized test scores are best at predicting your socioeconomic status rather than your ability to do something well. Why then would schools require this useless exam?

For nearly 100 years, premedical students everywhere have been taking the MCAT exam. In particular, the MCAT gives medical schools a means to compare two students from two different schools. While many factors contribute to your GPA (e.g. your performance, the professor, a grading curve, your mood that semester—

your professor's mood that semester), the MCAT provides an opportunity to compare people based on a standardized measure—a standardized exam score.

Some studies suggest the MCAT is good for predicting two things: your performance during the first two years of medical school and whether you will pass the first step of the United States Medical Licensing Exam (USMLE). Again, the exam does not predict whether you will be a good physician, it just predicts whether you will be able to pass Step 1. According to the AAMC's "Using MCAT Data in 2010 Selection," students who received a 30 or above on the MCAT had a 90% or better pass rate on USML Step 1.

Of all applicants who took the MCAT in 2009, the average total MCAT score was a 24.9 with a standard deviation of 6.4. The mean for each individual section ranged from an 8.0 to 8.7 with biological sciences having the highest mean (8.7). There were significant differences in total MCAT score based on race/ethnicity: the mean for Black or African Americans was 19.8; the mean for Native Hawaiian or Pacific Islanders was 21.1; the mean for Hispanic or Latinos was 21.5; the mean for American Indians or Alaskan Natives was 23.4; the mean for Asians was 25.9; the mean for Whites was 26.1.

A few medical schools have created pipeline programs for undergraduate students who want to become physicians. One such school is my very own medical school, the Icahn School of Medicine at Mount Sinai. These pipeline programs accept students while they are still in college often based on SAT scores, GPA, an essay and an interview, but do not require the MCAT. That's right. Groups of undergraduates are being accepted to medical school without the MCAT.

Once they get to medical school, most do fine! This is proof the MCAT is useless. However, since not all schools are ready to revamp the premedical curriculum and admissions requirements, most of you will take the MCAT. I had to take the MCAT too as I was accepted to my medical school via the traditional route.

Some believe that the MCAT is more important than your GPA. While it's very difficult to confirm whether this is true or not, I can tell you for certain that a good MCAT score will not hurt your chances of being accepted to medical school. On the other hand, a poor MCAT score will work against you. That being said, there are countless stories of students with less than stellar MCAT scores being accepted to medical school; some are at the end of this book.

Even though it may seem arbitrary at times, the truth is that most medical schools require you to take the MCAT. So you have to do it. No buts about it. So why not do all you can to do well?

Familiarize Yourself with the Exam

As with anything else, it's never too early to think about the MCAT. As a freshman, you can at least start to familiarize yourself with the structure of the exam. When is the exam offered? How much does it cost? How many sections are there? How many questions per section? How much time for each section? How much break time do you get in between each section? What subjects are covered on the exam? How is it scored?

The MCAT Basics

The MCAT was created by the Association of American Medical Colleges (AAMC). Get familiar with this acronym as the AAMC also hosts the American

Medical College Application Service (AMCAS). The current version of the MCAT covers general biology, general chemistry, organic chemistry, physics and verbal reasoning. General chemistry and physics are together in one section—the physical sciences (PS) section. Verbal reasoning (VR) is in a separate section, on its own. The last graded section is the biological sciences (BS) section which includes general biology and organic chemistry.

There is also a fourth section—a trial section. This trial section is completely voluntary as the makers of the exam, the AAMC, did away with the writing section and are preparing to roll out a new version of the MCAT in the year 2015. For each of the first three sections I mentioned, the highest score you can get on each is 15 for a total of 45 points. The trial section does not contribute to your score.

The entire exam takes approximately five hours. The PS and BS sections are each 70 minutes long and contain 52 questions each; the VR section is 60 minutes long and has 40 questions. The trial section has 32 questions and takes 45 minutes (but remember it's optional). In between each section, you can take a ten minute-long break.

The exam uses a combination of passage-based and "discrete" or independent questions not based on a passage. Passage-based questions require you to read a passage first before answering the questions. Discrete questions test your knowledge of specific scientific concepts and are not related to a passage. The VR section is the only section that is entirely passage-based.

For those of you who will not take the exam until 2015 or beyond, you will take an entirely new version of the MCAT. The new exam tests the same natural science subjects but also tests biochemistry. There is a brand new section called Psychological, Social and Biological

Foundations of Behavior which includes biology, sociology and psychology. Each section will have 67 questions and last 95 minutes except for the new and improved verbal reasoning section. The new verbal reasoning section is called Critical Analysis and Reasoning Skills, has 60 questions, and lasts 90 minutes. Therefore there will be a total of four graded sections for a total possible score of 60 instead of the old 45.

Schedule, Cost and Registration

The MCAT exam is offered at least once per month from January through September. On some days, the exam will be offered twice (once in the morning and once in the afternoon). As of 2013, it costs $270 to register.

Some students may be eligible for the Fee Assistance Program (FAP). Acceptance to FAP is based on you and your parent's financial information. As of 2013, applicants whose 2012 total family income is 300 percent or less of the 2012 poverty level for their family size are eligible for FAP. According to the Health and Human Services (HHS) 2011 Poverty Guidelines, the poverty level for a family of four is $22,350. This means a student from a family of four with a combined income of $67,050 or less would be eligible for FAP. See the Resource List for links to the FAP and HHS websites.

The most important features of FAP are reduced cost of MCAT registration, free medical school guidebook called the Medical School Admissions Requirements (MSAR) and application to up to 14 schools for free with AMCAS. You can only receive assistance from FAP up to five times throughout your life and you cannot receive assistance retroactively. This means you can immediately begin to think about when you will take the MCAT, when you will apply to medical school and you should read about FAP eligibility requirements and deadlines early on.

All of this information is available on the test-maker's website. See the Resource Page for more information. By familiarizing yourself with the exam early on, you are giving yourself a studying advantage. You will feel more comfortable beginning to study when it is actually time to do so. You are eliminating a huge potential for unnecessary anxiety.

Med-MAR

The Medical Minority Applicant Registry (Med-MAR) was created to enhance admissions opportunities for groups historically underrepresented in medicine, as described on the AAMC's Med-MAR website (see the Resource List). US citizens or permanent residents who will take the MCAT and identify as African American/Black, Hispanic/Latino, American Indian/Alaska Native or Native Hawaiian/Pacific Islander or are economically disadvantaged are eligible for Med-MAR. Med-MAR automatically forwards biographical information and your MCAT score to all admissions offices of AAMC-member medical schools interested in increasing diversity. If you are an underrepresented minority or economically disadvantaged, definitely join Med-MAR when you register for the MCAT.

Follow Along

If you really want to have an advantage, you can buy a used MCAT review book during your first year of college. See the Resource List for some suggestions. As you complete each course relevant to the exam, look at the review book to see which topics from the course the MCAT most emphasizes.

While it is not necessary (and there are other activities you can do to strengthen your AMCAS application), you can begin to study for sections of the MCAT as you finish the relevant coursework. You do not have be hardcore and study religiously. Simply glance over the review to get a feel for the content tested. When you are a year or two away from taking the exam, you can begin to answer questions here and there to get used to the way things are asked on the exam.

Setting a Realistic Goal

Do not plan to take the MCAT until you have taken all of the necessary coursework. For example, you should complete general biology, general chemistry, organic chemistry, physics and possibly even biochemistry before you take the exam. You will have also wanted to complete at least one social science course like psychology or sociology. Keep in mind that many people do not follow this rule. Some of these people do fine on the exam. I'm all about ensuring you do as well as possible. Wait to complete your coursework first, even if that means that you apply to medical school during your last year of college or after graduation instead of your junior year of college.

Some people will tell you to aim for a perfect score. This is a nice thought but most people will not earn a perfect score. You need to set a realistic goal. You must at least perform at or above the national average. The higher the better. However, all you need is a score that will allow you to be a successful applicant. This number is different for everyone. For example, if you have a weak GPA you should aim for a higher MCAT score. If you have a great

GPA, wonderful extracurricular and clinical experiences then you do not need to get a 40 out of 45 on the MCAT.

You also need to think about which medical schools you want to attend. Even though the MCAT is not a great measure of what type of physician you will become, more "prestigious" schools will have a higher MCAT average for their most recently accepted class. Try to aim close to the school's average MCAT score but remember that an average is just an average.

Some accepted students performed above the average and some below the average. A safe score is 30 or above out of 45 since according to the AAMC, you are more likely to pass USMLE Step 1, as previously mentioned. It's also better to be as well-rounded as possible: a 14 on one section and 8 on the other two sections is bad news. It's better to have an even 10 in each section. However, please remember that the MCAT is not everything. At the end of this book you will find countless stories of students who were admitted to medical school with an MCAT score lower than a 30.

Finally Time to Start Studying

To enroll in a prep course or not to enroll in a prep course, that is the question. That is a question only you can answer. It all comes down to self-awareness. For many, a prep course is absolutely essential and for others it's a big waste of time.

I took a prep course because I'm a person who enjoys structure. The course had its own syllabus which I used to keep myself on track. The only downfall was that my course only met once a week for several months. In hindsight it would have been much better to have taken a course that met several times per week for just a few months. Intense study for a shorter duration of time is better than dragging it out over six months. However, you may elect to study both before and after the prep course as well.

The other great thing about my prep course was that I had a fabulous instructor. He had a wonderful knack for explaining things in a simple and elegant way that stuck in my mind. To be honest, the instructor is what determines whether the course will be meaningful or not. Be sure to ask around (ask friends and older students) whether they know of any good MCAT instructors and see if you can enroll that instructor's course.

The other great thing about the prep course I took was free access to AAMC practice MCATs. Most prep course companies have their own practice tests to take which is essential. The company's practice tests were good because after each test, I received a report that highlighted my strengths and weaknesses. I was able to tailor my studying accordingly. However, these company practice tests are not exactly like the real thing. The AAMC practice exams are actually formerly-administered tests so they are as realistic as it can get. Keep in mind that if you do not take a prep course, you can still purchase AAMC practice tests on your own for $35 each as of 2013.

How to Actually Study

Studying for the MCAT is like preparing to run a marathon. Athletes don't just show up on the day of the race ready to go. They train for months leading up to race. Athletes may combine cardio, strength training and endurance training in preparation for the race. They don't just physically train, they also eat right and get enough rest; they also train their minds. As a premedical student you need to study material and take practice tests, but you also need to eat right, sleep enough and envision yourself succeeding on the test day. You can do it. Remember, the MCAT is just an exam. While it is important for admission to medical school, that is all it is good for!

First thing's first. Take a practice test to see what your baseline MCAT score would be. Certain test prep companies offer practice MCATs for free. Don't study for the practice test. Just take it, and don't be alarmed by your score. Most people who take the practice MCAT cold will score low. That's okay. That is the point.

Even if you do not enroll in a formal prep course, I highly recommend buying a review book. You cannot study for the MCAT without professionally prepared review material. Some of the more popular review companies include Kaplan, Princeton Review and Examkrackers. Some people think they can review science content from their college textbooks. This is a mistake! Your text books cover way more information than is required for the MCAT. If you do not understand something that is written in the review book, you can always turn to your text book for additional information. However, text books should not be your primary source. The review book will highlight high-yield concepts often tested on the MCAT and will provide you with summary tables and figures (saving you time)!

Verbal Reasoning

I like to use the VR score as a measure of your potential on the MCAT. If you have low science scores but a high VR score, this means you probably need to review more science content. Then you can do just as well on the sciences as you did in VR. Doing well on VR means that you probably know how to navigate the tricky things about standardized exams (e.g. time constraints, question format). However, this rule does not apply if English is not your first language. In this case, your VR score may or may not be your lowest score.

Prepare to read a lot and broadly in preparation for the VR section. I read the NY Times every day (not just the Science Times) and also read Scientific American. Any reputable newspaper will do. This will help you on the VR section and during your medical school interview (more on this later). Every time you come across a word you don't understand, look it up. You may also consider taking a critical reading or philosophy class to help you learn to read critically.

What does it mean to read critically? Reading critically requires you to focus on what the author is trying to accomplish with each paragraph as you read. Instead of becoming wrapped up in the words written on the page or the story, think critically about each passage or news article you read. What is the author's main point? What is the main idea? What is the author's purpose? Is the author trying to inform or persuade you? What is the author's opinion on the issue being described? Pay special attention to transition words like "however," "although," or "furthermore" as these will provide insight into what the author is doing with his words.

Get into the habit of writing a 3-5 word "summary" of each paragraph. For example, you may write "author disagrees w/ current law" next to one paragraph and "examples of ad results" next to another paragraph. The only person who has to understand this summary is you. Be concise so that you save time but don't be so vague that the summaries are meaningless to you. Also, underline transition words. The point of writing paragraph summaries and underlining transition words is to define the structure of the passage; how it is written rather than what is written. By writing paragraph summaries, it will be easier for you to answer the questions based on the passage without actually going back and rereading the entire thing (a huge waste of time).

Science Sections

As you read your review book, complete all the assignments and questions within the book as you go along (this applies for VR too). I also found it helpful to make flash cards for important science concepts. Computer programs such as Anki, will help you organize and review electronic flashcards if handwriting flashcards seems too time consuming. Another thing I would highly recommend is using Examkrackers 1001 questions/passage series. I have no conflicts of interest to disclose, and I'm simply naming Examkrackers because this series is truly one of a kind. They have EK 1001 books for each subject; in addition to using all of my prep course material, I used EK 1001 series to drill myself with questions for at least 30 minutes a day.

When you feel as though you're done reviewing content, take another practice test. If you are not enrolled in a prep course or do not have access to practice tests, I highly recommend that you purchase AAMC practice exams. Try to save your AAMC practice tests for the end of your study regimen (more on this later). If you did very well on your first practice test you may not see a big increase in your score for the second practice exam. However, the lower your original score the greater the potential for a large increase. For example, if you got a 15 in total on the first practice exam it will be easier to see a score increase than if you got a 30 the first time around.

At the end of this second practice test, it is absolutely imperative that you review each question. Whether you got a question right or wrong, review it. If you got it right, were you guessing or did you actually know the answer? If you got the question wrong, why did you get it wrong? Were you simply short on time? Did you misread the question or answer choices? Did you just not know the concept? What could be changed about the question so that you would have gotten it correct? If you are mostly happy with your second practice test score, you may be ready to move from content review to an intense practice test training period.

40 Days Before the Exam

I do not take credit for the following: my MCAT instructor helped me come up with a study schedule that I nicknamed "40 Days Before." 40 Days Before requires you to study more intensely 40 days before your exam. From my baseline practice exam to my second or third practice exam, my score jumped about eight points. Then I plateaued at a score with which I was not happy. 40 Days Before gave me the extra five-point boost I needed just a week before the real MCAT.

So what is 40 Days Before? It varies depending on how many practice exams you have left to complete. For forty days, you will take practice exams and will not review any content. You should time each exam and take your test in a quiet area, just like the real thing. You will start of slowly, work up to an intense week of practice exams and then rest for a week just before your real exam.

You should only do this when you're done reviewing content. If you're not done reviewing content forty days before your real exam, then you should reschedule your exam date. Push it back by a month or two. Don't be afraid to push back your exam—it's better to knock it out of the park the first time around than to have to retake the MCAT.

The practice test schedule is as follows and is completely customizable:

40 days before exam	1st AAMC practice test
30 days before exam	2nd AAMC practice test
21 days before exam	3rd AAMC practice test
17 days before exam	4th AAMC practice test
13 days before exam	5th AAMC practice test
11 days before exam	6th AAMC practice test
9 days before exam	7th AAMC practice test
7 days before exam	RELAX!

After each exam you must, must, must review each and every single question. You must review every single question! **You must review every single question!** Got it? Part of the review process may also include going back to your review book or textbook for clarity on a topic.

If you find yourself turning to your review book or textbook often, then you probably began 40 Days Before too early and need to go back to reviewing content. 40 Days Before is supposed to help you build endurance and overcome the format of the exam, as each practice exam is similar to the real thing and timed. You should not be using 40 Days Before if you still need to review content.

You are supposed to rest during the week leading up to your exam because, let's face it, if you don't know it a week before the exam you will not learn it in a week. However, I was not comfortable doing nothing for an entire week. To keep my mind in shape, I did one hour per day of EK 1001 series. This was useful for me. It boosted my confidence. If you think drilling yourself with questions will stress you out, then don't do it. You want to be as comfortable and well-rested as possible during the week leading up to your exam. You definitely should not review any more content or take any more practice tests during the final week. You don't want to psych yourself out a week before your exam in the event that you realize you don't know a topic as well as you had hoped.

External Factors

During one of my interviews, I was asked how I studied for the MCAT. I went off on a five minute rant about all of the study techniques I used only to be interrupted by my interviewer. "Were you working and going to school while you studied?" he asked. He just wanted to know how many things I juggled in addition to studying for the MCAT.

The MCAT is important for admission to medical school so it is important to do as well as you can. However, you should also realize that medical school is just as intense as studying for the MCAT and probably more so. In medical school you will also take high-stakes exams and have to juggle a number of things. My interviewer asked me that question to gain some insight into my MCAT score and to determine whether I am capable of handling the workload in medical school.

Some students decide to take off from work and school to study for the exam. If this is what you need to do in order to do well on the MCAT, fine. It is okay to lighten your workload and make the MCAT a priority. However, do not fall into the trap of studying, studying, studying, postponing your exam, studying, studying, studying, postpone your exam again, studying, studying...you get the idea. I've seen many students allow the MCAT to take over their life and this is just wrong. You'll go insane! It is true that the MCAT will take over your life for a short while as you study intensely and during 40 Days Before, but you should not be skipping school and work for a year to take the MCAT.

At some point you have to just take the exam. While you don't want to rush, you also need to be honest with yourself: if you have not seen your score increase in months, then you are either ready to take the exam or need to seriously reconsider the way in which you are studying.

Bombed It...Now What?

If you are asking yourself this question, first define "bombed." Did you miss your target score by a point or two? Did you do terribly in one section and great in the others? Did you completely fall way below your target score or below the national average? Depending on your answer to these questions, you may reconsider taking the exam...or not.

Every student's situation is different. Your MCAT score is just one piece of your medical school application and so when considering to retake it, you have to consider your entire AMCAS application (more on

AMCAS later). If you missed your target score by a point or two, you probably should not retake the exam. If you did well in most sections but poorly in others, you need to meet with a mentor or advisor to determine whether it is in your best interest to retake the exam or not. If you did poorly on the VR section because of a language issue, it may be better to discuss your language issue somewhere else on your application rather than retake the entire exam. The combination of MCAT score, GPA, extracurricular activities and personal statements are limitless, so there is no one solution for everyone.

There is one thing that applies to everyone. Medical schools can see your MCAT score, every time you take it. Therefore, you should not make the decision to retake the exam without first seriously reflecting on your entire MCAT experience. You don't want to take an exam three times and not increase your score at all or worse, decrease your score. In order to ensure that your score will improve, you need to seriously evaluate what happened the first time around.

The first thing to ask yourself is what went wrong? Did your nerves get the best of you? If so, then retaking the exam may or may not help. You will either overcome your test anxiety during the second MCAT because you've seen the real exam once before, or you will feel pressure to do better the second time around which could send your test anxiety through the roof. Only you can decide which scenario describes you best.

If it was not a matter of nerves or test anxiety, were you simply unprepared? Did you take the exam despite disappointing practice test scores? The trickiest thing about the MCAT is that there is no one size fits all study solution. You must find a balance between preparing to take the exam without allowing it to overcome your life. Sometimes students focus too much on the latter and end up taking it too early (despite warning signs telling them to postpone the exam). If this is what happened to you, then you will need to study more before retaking the exam.

If you felt completely prepared, did not have test anxiety, did not experience some other unusual life event at the time of your exam yet still bombed it, then you need to reevaluate your study technique. At this point, it may be useful to consult a professional test preparation company, your premedical advisor, an MCAT tutor or other person who knows how to effectively counsel students in this situation. You could be missing one little thing that is preventing you from improving your score or you could be in need of an entire study overhaul.

MCAT: Final Word

As with most things in life, the MCAT is very personal. Your target score, study method and performance should be individualized. It is important for you to be self-aware and use your self-awareness along with study materials and maybe even professional help to design and execute a study method that works for you. Whether you take time off from school or work is entirely your decision. How much time you spend studying for the MCAT is entirely up to you as well. Whether you take the MCAT a second or third time is also your decision. Please read the Stories for Inspiration at the end of this book to learn about other's stories.

10 AMCAS

So, you've chosen a major, worked hard in college, participated in extracurricular activities, asked for letters of recommendation, spent your summers in a productive way, took the MCAT and now you're ready to apply to medical school! Now it's all about AMCAS.

The Association of American Medical Colleges (AAMC) is in charge of AMCAS. AMCAS stands for the American Medical College Application Service. As stated on the AMCAS website, AMCAS is "a centralized application processing service that is only available to applicants to the first-year entering classes at participating U.S. medical schools. Most medical schools use AMCAS as the primary application method." By the end of your application cycle, admissions committees across the nation may know you better than your best friend knows you. Get ready to get personal. When you complete your AMCAS application, it automatically gets forwarded to the schools you select. There are several parts to the

AMCAS application; each of them will be discussed. But first...

Staying Organized

You must remain organized throughout the entire application process. Most schools require you to submit a primary application via AMCAS, a secondary application, supporting documents (e.g. passport photo or updated transcript) and finally interview with the school—that's a lot! You want to make sure that you do not miss any deadlines and follow up on everything.

I would highly recommend creating a spreadsheet. On the left-hand side list every school to which you want to apply. In subsequent columns, list whether or not you have completed the primary application, submitted the application, or the application has been processed. In the next column, you will list the status of the secondary application for each school (e.g. received, completed, submitted, or processed). You will then do the same thing for any application fees, supporting documents, interviews, thank you notes (more on this later) and finally, the final status of your application (accepted, waitlisted, or rejected). Now, back to AMCAS...

Identifying Information and Contact Information

These first few sections are very self-explanatory. You will input your basic identifying information (e.g. name, date of birth, birthplace, primary language etc.) and your contact information.

Biographic Information

Here you will identify biographical information including language spoken, legal residence, race and ethnicity.

Childhood Information

In this section you will list your primary childhood residence. You will provide information about your family's financial situation, and you can report whether you consider yourself underserved. To determine if you are underserved, AMCAS asks, "Do you believe, based on your own experiences or the experiences of family and friends that the area in which you grew up was inadequately served by the available health care professionals? Were there enough physicians, nurses, hospitals, clinics, and other health care service providers?"

Disadvantaged Statement

If you believe you are disadvantaged, you will check a box and a form will appear in which you will write your disadvantaged statement. But how do you know if you are disadvantaged? According to U.S. News and World Report, there are three reasons for which you can designate yourself as disadvantaged on AMCAS: if you chose to identify as underserved in the previous section; if a situation in your immediate family negatively influenced your educational opportunities or social circumstances; you received aid from assistance programs such as

Supplemental Nutrition Assistance Program, Medicaid, free school lunch etc.

While being disadvantaged by definition sets you back in life, it is an advantage to be disadvantaged when you apply to medical schools. This is because many medical schools will consider your disadvantaged status as they review the rest of your application. If you had to learn English as a second language, it may have had an impact on your MCAT score. If you had to work to support your family while you were in school, it may have had an impact on your grades. Please remember that not all schools weigh your disadvantaged status in the same way.

While it may be tempting, please do not lie about your disadvantaged status in an attempt to get "extra points" on your application. Anything you put in your application is fair game during a medical school interview. If medical schools don't figure out you're lying by then (or during the interview itself), they will probably find out when you submit tax forms to apply for financial aid. In any case, lying will certainly buy you rejections at all the schools to which you applied. Admissions committees at different schools often talk to each other.

If you identify as disadvantaged, your statement is just as important as your personal statement. The only difference is that your disadvantaged statement has to be to the point without any fluff—there just isn't any room to write a long essay. Here are examples of entire disadvantaged statements from REAL applications:

My family and I have always struggled financially - in China and in the United States. The thought of becoming a physician while growing up in China was merely a dream because of my family's financial and social status. I am extremely thankful to have the opportunity here in the United States. I had to work in order to pay for tuition and expenses to earn a college degree. I am the first person in my family to graduate from college and I would like to become a physician so I can work in underserved communities like my own. No one in my family has medical insurance and I know many people in my community cannot afford it. As a result, members of my family and community have often gone without routine health care.

I grew up in a rural area in a country with inadequate healthcare. The shortage of healthcare providers had an effect on me, my family, and the entire community. My siblings and I came to the United States in 1992 and lived with only our mother, as my father died a few years ago. We have been living in Brooklyn, in a poverty-stricken area overrun with crime, violence, drugs and danger. English is not my first language and I had to learn the language and assimilate into a new culture when we first moved to New York. I have also had to work to support myself since college began.

I grew up in the Bronx, NY. My parents never attended college. My father was a drug addict and my parents divorced when I was a child. My mother suffered from a stroke which left her unable to work. Throughout my life, my family received aid from government assistance programs such as food stamps, Medicaid and free school meals.

Another very important rule to follow while writing your disadvantaged statement is to remain positive. At times what you write will paint a grim picture, but don't exaggerate. Make sure that in the disadvantaged statement or somewhere else in your application you describe how you overcame that adversity. Where you choose to discuss overcoming adversity will depend on how much room you have left in your disadvantaged statement.

Parents, Guardians, Siblings, Additional Applicant Information

In this section, you will provide biographical information about your parents, guardians and siblings. You will also disclose sensitive information such as felony convictions, misdemeanors, suspension or expulsion from school etc.

Academic Record and Standardized Test Scores

In this section you will list each course name, course number, number of credits for the course and the course letter grade for all courses you have taken as an undergraduate, post-baccalaureate, or graduate student; you will also list the institution at which you completed the credits. You have an opportunity to list College Level Examination Program (CLEP) or advanced placement (AP) credits as well.

In addition to inputting your coursework for the application, you are also required to submit an official transcript to AMCAS. Once your application is processed AMCAS will generate a GPA for you for "BCPM" or biology, chemistry, physics and math (also known as your science GPA). AMCAS will also generate an "AO" or all other GPA, and finally a total GPA. AMCAS will also break down your GPA by class standing (i.e. freshman, sophomore, junior or senior) and then list a cumulative GPA.

Sometimes there can be a discrepancy between your official transcript GPA and the AMCAS GPA. This is most often because AMCAS treats grades of A+ the same as A. Another common reason why a discrepancy may occur is because you may have failed a course and repeated it. Some colleges will not include the original F in your GPA, however, AMCAS does. In any case, AMCAS has the final word. Medical schools will use the information listed on your AMCAS application.

Standardized exam scores, such as your MCAT results, will also be automatically uploaded to AMCAS (you don't have to worry about it). You can also list an additional MCAT intent date for the year if you have already registered to take the MCAT again. Other test scores can be included on AMCAS as well (e.g. GRE, DAT, PCAT) if you took other standardized exams.

Experiences

You can add up to 15 experiences. Experiences include actual extracurricular activities, research, honors and awards, employment, publications, shadowing and other clinical experiences, even hobbies. There are a few rules to follow when it comes to deciding which experiences to include in AMCAS.

First, you may have more than 15 experiences. If this is the case, choose the experiences that were most meaningful to you or that are the most prestigious. You also want to make sure you present a diverse array of experiences. Don't just list 15 times in which you shadowed a physician. The following is an example of how to organize your experiences. I have organized them by category, similar to those AMCAS asks you to designate for each experience:

Honors/Awards/Recognition
- Graduate of the Year
- Molecular Biology Research Award
- Graduating Senior Scholarship
- Science Undergraduate Fellowship
- Phi Beta Kappa

Publications
- Premedical Club Newsletter

Research/Lab
- Undergraduate thesis work

Community Service/Volunteer-medical
- Medical Assistant
- Emergency Department Volunteer

Community Service/Volunteer-non-medical
- Mentor
- Senior Citizen Center Volunteer

Paid Employment-military
- none

Paid Employment-non-military
- Tutor
- The Gap

Other
- *Friendly's*
- *none*

Ensuring that you present a diverse array of experiences is not the only rule. If you have less than 15 experiences, that is okay. Do not feel obligated to fill all 15 spaces. In doing so, you may start to pick and choose experiences that didn't mean much to you or random experiences that don't add to your story (e.g. remember that one time you randomly shadowed a doctor for one hour?). You don't need to fill space.

Finally, we get to the meat of the experiences section: actually writing about your experiences. For each entry you will have to list the following: experience type; experience name; dates; hours; contact person's name and title; contact person's email; contact person's phone number; organization name; city/state/country; experience description. There is also an option to designate a particular experience as "most meaningful." You can choose up to three most meaningful experiences and this will give you extra space to write about each one.

Treat each experience essay like a mini personal statement. All of the same rules apply about sticking to good mechanics of writing. Only this time, the focus of what you write should be a description of your role and duties or information about the award or honor. It will be easiest to show you a few examples.

The following three experiences come from my very own AMCAS application:

Experience Type: Publication
Experience Name: POZ Magazine/Treatment Issues
Contact Name and Title: X
Contact email: Y
Contact Phone Number: Z
Organization Name: Gay Men's Health Crisis (GMHC)
City/State/Country: New York/NY/United States of America
Dates: 12/2009
Hours: n/a
Most Meaningful Experience: No
Experience Description: I wrote the article called "Gender inequality and corrective rape of women who have sex with women," during my time as a Public Policy Fellow at GMHC. This article focused on the disturbing phenomenon of "corrective rape" and how it contributes to the spread of HIV/AIDS in Africa (the United States is discussed as well). The article was published in print in POZ Magazine's quarterly publication "Treatment Issues," and can be found online at: http://www.poz.com/pdfs/gmhc_treatmentissues_2009_12.pdf

Experience Type: Honors/Awards/Recognitions
Experience Name: Golden Key International Honor Society
Contact Name and Title: X
Contact email: Y
Contact Phone Number: Z
Organization Name: The City University of New York

City/State/Country: New York/NY/United States of America
Dates: 05/2010
Hours: n/a
Most Meaningful Experience: No
Experience Description: Senior undergraduate students inducted into this honor society are in the top 15% of their class.

Experience Type: Community Service/Volunteer-non-medical
Experience Name: Minority Association of Premedical Students (MAPS)
Contact Name and Title: X
Contact email: Y
Contact Phone Number: Z
Organization Name: The City University of New York
City/State/Country: New York/NY/United States of America
Dates: 09/2006-06/2011
Hours: 6/week
Most Meaningful Experience: Yes
Experience Description: MAPS is the undergraduate branch of the Student National Medical Association (SNMA). I became a member of the City College chapter in 2006. In 2008, I became Secretary and in 2009, I became President. I began my second term as President in 2010. During my three years on the executive board I developed and coordinated professional development seminars for members, fundraisers, and community service events for the Harlem community. I served as prime coordinator of an annual health fair that serves over 200 people from the Harlem and Washington Heights communities.

Most Meaningful Experience Remarks: The first time I heard "health disparities" was when I became a MAPS member. Prior to joining MAPS I had only known about health disparities from first-hand accounts in my neighborhood and never put a name to the health inequities I witnessed. Through MAPS I not only became interested in health disparities but also started to look at public health in a more critical way. I also learned about osteopathic medicine as a MAPS member and was able to explore what the profession entailed, further solidifying my hopes of becoming an allopathic physician.

MAPS inspired me and as I served in various leadership positions, I had an opportunity to see how MAPS functions at the national level in tandem with the SNMA. I also attended the annual MAPS/SNMA regional and national conferences. I was able to hone in on my leadership skills, and devoted immense amounts of my time and energy to serving other students and the Harlem community. Our chapter hosts an annual health fair and during my time as president I was able to increase attendance from 9 to over 200 community members. I also helped our chapter be named 2011 National MAPS Chapter of the Year for the first time. MAPS helped shape the context in which I view medicine and further strengthened my desire to become a physician.

From these examples, you can see that some experiences require a detailed explanation (e.g. publications) while others require a very short description (e.g. honor society). Additionally, you can see that you are allowed to write a lot (almost an entire essay) for "most meaningful experiences." For your most meaningful experiences, be prepared to truly demonstrate why the experience was so meaningful to you.

Personal Comments

This is where your personal statement will be entered.

Letters of Evaluation/Recommendation

You will list contact information for your recommenders and/or premedical committee/advisor. The recommenders will submit their letters to AMCAS on their own.

Designated Programs

Here you will select the schools to which you want your AMCAS application forwarded. You can select as many as you like. In 2013, the AMCAS processing fee was $160 and includes one medical school designation; each additional medical school to which you apply will cost $35 each.

It is very important to apply to a wide range of programs. There is no such thing as a "safety" school when it comes to medical school admissions. However, you can get an idea of how competitive a school is based on admissions statistics and statistics for its most recently accepted first-year class. These statistics are often posted on the school's website and in the MSAR. The MSAR has at least one page dedicated to every school that chose to submit information; the page includes information about application fees, previously accepted incoming class statistics, special programs, diversity statistics, tuition etc.

You should always apply to all of your state schools. Apply to some "mid-level" schools and to some "reach" schools. The definition of "mid-level" or "reach" is different for each applicant. You can decide what a reasonable choice is based on your GPA, extracurricular activities, MCAT score and essay. However, please, please, please keep in mind that you never know exactly what medical schools want. Even if a school may seem out of your reach, it may be worth applying to it anyway to see what happens, especially if you're very interested in attending that particular school.

Also, many people who are supposed to advise you (premed advisors, mentors, parents, family etc.) are sometimes the people who tell you that you cannot achieve something. There are plenty of reasons why someone may believe you should not become a doctor: your GPA is too low; you have too many W's on your transcript; you should work and earn money instead incur debt from medical school; you will never be able to afford medical school; you should become a nurse instead to avoid the long training; you'll never fit in. While I hope this is not the case, you should have faith in yourself no matter what, and take everything you hear with a grain of salt. Just because your premed advisor thinks you will be rejected from a school doesn't mean that he or she is absolutely correct. Please read the Stories of Inspiration to learn about real students who beat all odds to be admitted to medical school.

Other AMCAS Tips

The application usually opens in June. Even if you don't have everything together, in June you can begin to input the information you do have prepared (e.g. biographical information). You can also ask your recommenders to submit their letters early, and you can submit your transcript. There is no need to wait for your MCAT score to be posted on AMCAS or your personal statement to be perfected. Start working on your AMCAS application as soon as you can, and enter the various components as they are ready to be entered.

It is important to submit your application early for two reasons. First, after you click "submit" the application must still be processed and go through the verification process to make sure everything you submitted (e.g. coursework) is accurate and true. Your recommendation letters, transcript and MCAT scores must also be received by AMCAS in order for your application to be considered complete. The earlier your application is submitted and eventually sent to the medical schools you chose, the better your chances are of being invited for an interview.

Many medical schools participate in what is called "rolling" admissions. This means that as they receive applications, they invite select applicants for interviews. Then, after a certain period of time following your interview you will know whether or not you've been accepted. In other words, you will not have to wait until the end of the admissions cycle to learn whether or not you've been accepted. Most schools that have rolling admissions make final decisions within weeks of interviewing you. This means that the earlier you apply, the more likely you are to be interviewed because the pool of applicants from which a school can choose to interview, may be relatively small or the school has not yet accepted that many applicants. The higher your chances are of acceptance. This means you have a higher chance of being selected.

This process is not true for all schools. Some schools will interview applicants throughout the entire admissions cycle and then notify every single applicant all at once on a certain day. They do not have rolling admissions. This way, these medical schools are able to make a decision only after everyone has been interviewed. This means a spot in the class won't be "wasted" on a less qualified applicant who was simply conscientious enough to submit his application early.

Finally, proofread your entire application. PROOFREAD YOUR APPLICATION! I cannot stress this enough. Print out a hard copy of your application and ask at least two people to proofread it. By the time you think you've finished your application, you will know each word so well that you may overlook typos, grammatical errors or problems with spelling and punctuation. It is absolutely necessary for at least two other people to proofread your application.

Your Electronic Alter Ego

Nowadays, grandparents are on Facebook and Twitter. More people than ever before have access to the internet and are using social media. Every day more and more social media sites are born. Despite its widespread use, you as a medical school applicant will have to seriously monitor what you put into cyber space.

For starters, you need a professional email address for your medical school application. SexyBaby123 simply won't do. You should choose something simple that uses your first and last name or initials with a combination of numbers (if necessary). You should also get into the habit of checking this email at least once a day as medical schools will send you very important information (e.g. interview invitations) via email.

Once you have a professional email address, you have to clean up your social media profiles. Remember that medical schools love any excuse to reject you because it helps them narrow down the applicant pool. It makes their job easier. No one is going to excuse even one misstep. This means you must start to think like an admissions committee member. Every time you're about to post a photo, status, tweet—whatever—ask yourself, "What would admissions think about this?" For example, you may be of legal drinking age and want to post a photo of yourself sipping wine at a sophisticated soiree. While this seems harmless, stop and ask yourself, "What would admissions think about this?" If you think for even just a second that someone, somewhere in the world can misinterpret your photo as unprofessional, then do not post it. The same applies for everything else related to the internet: blogs, status updates, posts, comments etc.

I know it may sound like you're being a phony, but you want to create an online personality that you would be proud to show to medical schools. For example, it is okay to post a link to an article you recently read. It's okay to keep a blog as long as you maintain your professionalism. It's okay to leave funny comments on your friend's pages as long as it does not make you look unprofessional. This means do not use profanity, do not comment on highly controversial topics that can be taken the wrong way, do not brag about how much alcohol you drank last night or how hung over you are…you get the idea. For the record, making your page "private" does not solve the issue; some software programs get around privacy settings and some medical schools use such programs.

Now you may be thinking to yourself "crap," as you recall that unprofessional photo lingering on your Facebook. No worries. Simply delete it. Or untag yourself. The sooner, the better. Or, if necessary, deactivate your account. My Facebook profile was not unprofessional but I just didn't want to go through the hassle of always trying to figure out what admissions committees might think about it…so I deleted it. Now, over two years later, my account is still deactivated. Social media can be a total time sink.

On the other hand, I do have a LinkedIn and Twitter profile, and I blog. Only I don't use these websites to comment on very personal things. For the most part, I use these websites to promote my projects, share thoughts about medical school or current events with others and to connect with other professionals. How you choose to use social media is entirely up to you, but choose wisely.

Finally, get into the habit of writing professional emails. Please do not use "lol," "u" instead of "you" or smiley faces. This is completely inappropriate for medical school correspondence. You should also learn to write a nicely worded email with proper formatting. For example:

Dear Mr. Soandso,

I hope this message finds you well! My name is X. I am a senior at University Y. I am writing to you to learn more about Program Z. I'm interested in Program Z because_____, and I would love to learn more about it from your perspective. Please let me know if you are available to speak on the phone or in person. I can be reached at 867-5309 or via email at this address. I look forward to hearing from you.

Sincerely,
X

Not every email has to follow this format word-for-word. You need to find a salutation with which you're comfortable and a way to conclude and sign the letter. This is often overlooked as people are used to replying to emails using their smart phones. You should always use proper English and spellcheck and reread your emails before you send them. Remember, admissions committees are just waiting for you to mess up. Everything you send to them (even emails) are put in your folder. An unprofessional email that makes you look careless can cause you to be rejected.

You should always include your contact information at the end of the email. Many email services will allow you to create a signature that automatically gets inserted into all of your emails. Your signature should include your name, title and contact information. For example, my current signature is:

Alexa M. Mieses, BS
MD/MPH Candidate, 2016
Clinic Manager, EHHOP Mental Health and Medical Clinics
Editor-in-Chief, the Rossi
Icahn School of Medicine at Mount Sinai
Cell Phone: xxx-xxx-xxxx
Website: www.AlexaMieses.com

Your electronic personality reflects on the real you and the decisions you make. Make sure you give yourself the best chance possible to be admitted to medical school. Don't sell yourself short by doing something silly online that can have serious effects in real life. Get a professional email, clean up your social media profiles, and always answer emails promptly and professionally.

11 SECONDARY APPLICATIONS

If you're filling out secondary applications, you're no longer in AMCAS territory. Medical schools send out secondary applications for different reasons. The only common prerequisite is that you submitted your primary application (AMCAS) to that particular school. Once you've applied to a school through AMCAS, they can send you a secondary application.

Some medical schools screen applicants before they send out secondary applications. This means that they will actually review your application and determine whether or not they want you to move on to the next step in the application process. Other schools send secondary applications to everyone who submitted a primary application via AMCAS, regardless of how desirable they are as candidates. In the MSAR, you can read about which method is used by your choice of medical schools.

No two secondary applications are exactly the same. You can tell right away which schools just want your secondary application fee (also known as, MONEY). These secondaries may actually ask you to repeat things you have already written on your AMCAS application or simply restate your biographical information. These applications don't tell the admissions committees anything new about you but you must complete it to be considered for an interview.

The other type of secondary essay is actually useful. You may be asked to include a photo. DO NOT TRY TO STAND OUT IN THIS PHOTO! Take a normal passport photo, wearing professional dress, with a warm facial expression. Submitting a photo dressed as Santa Claus or half naked are absolute no-no's (trust me it has happened). These are not headshots—no need for a seductive smile or tons of make up or photo effects. Keep it simple and professional. Also, to really be safe, remove any excessive or radical piercings and cover tattoos—you never know if someone will judge you because of it.

Aside from a photo, most secondaries will also ask you to include your biographical information, and ask at least one other essay question. These secondary essays may allow you to explain a poor grade, what you did with your gap year or what class you enjoyed most. Another common secondary essay question asks you to describe why you want to attend school X. The secondary essays may ask you ethical questions or questions to further elucidate how you view medicine.

When you write your secondary essays think about what medical schools want to hear. Although you cannot lie on your application, you can frame things in a way that will work in your favor. For example, if you are asked to discuss your favorite class, make sure you don't give a silly reason like "the professor was a really easy grader." If you are asked to discuss what it means to be a physician don't say "it means that I will always have a job and earn enough money." Both of the examples I gave may be true but you need to convey professionalism, maturity and altruism at all times. Here are examples of secondary essay prompts:

1. *What aspects of the field of medicine most intrigue you and describe how they will influence your medical practice. (1 page or less)*
2. *Do you wish to include any comments (in addition to those already provided in your AMCAS application) to the Admissions Committee at X University School of Medicine? (1000 characters or less)*
3. *Have you taken or are you planning to take time off between college graduation and medical school matriculation? (1 page or less)*
4. *Tell us about a difficult or challenging situation you have encountered and how you dealt with it. In your response, identify both the coping skills you called upon to resolve the dilemma, and the support person (s) from whom you sought advice. (1000 words or less)*
5. *Have you been nominated for or received an award from any state, regional or national organization?*
6. *Describe an obstacle you have overcome and how it has defined you. (1 page or less)*

7. *Please explain your reasons for applying to the X School of Medicine and limit your response to 1,000 characters.*
8. *Our mission statement is an expression of our core purpose and educational philosophy. Please reflect on its content and write an essay describing why you see yourself as a great "fit" for X. (1000 words or less)*
9. *Describe an extracurricular experience you have had that will help you become a compassionate physician and explain why. (1 page or less)*
10. *If you are not attending college during the current academic year, what are your plans? Please limit your statement to less than 200 words.*

You want to make sure your essay questions are great before you submit the secondary essay. However, you do not need to give them as much attention as you did your personal statement. The longer you take to submit your secondary essays, the longer it will take for you to be invited for an interview. As always, you need to find the right balance between producing a good essay and not taking forever to write it. You don't want to delay your application. You also don't want to send in an essay that will jeopardize your candidacy.

Make sure that if they give you an opportunity to write additional comments, you take advantage of it. Don't ever leave a question (such as question #2) blank, unless it does not apply to you. Even if all you do is reiterate your interest in the school, answer the question (unless you already reiterated your interest in the school in another secondary application question for the same school).

The rules for writing a good personal statement still apply. Try to catch your reader's attention without going overboard. PROOFREAD your essays. PROOFREAD YOUR ESSAYS! I cannot stress this enough. If you are writing about a challenge or obstacle make sure you talk about how you overcame it. What did you learn? How did you overcome it? Who was your support system? Try to put a positive spin on everything you write and don't ever blame other people for your problems—especially not academic problems. There is one very important difference between secondary essays and your personal statement. Some secondary essay questions will be very straight forward with a limited maximum word length. In this case, you must be as straightforward as possible (similar to a disadvantaged statement).

You also need to be completely honest in your secondary applications. Do not lie about anything. Don't even exaggerate. Medical school admissions committees have a way of finding out the truth, and are just waiting for you to mess up so that they can reject you and move on to the next application. Do not give them a reason to dismiss you. Be positive and honest. Here are some real examples of secondary essays:

> *If the following statement is true, please explain: I have received at least one F during my undergraduate career.*
>
> In freshman year, I failed pre-calculus. I overcame many obstacles during high school (for example, a personal injury and severe bout of infectious mononucleosis) which interfered with my preparation in several classes, but especially math. During freshman year

of college, I was also working full-time which interfered with studying. I did not give pre-calculus the time it required and consequently failed. However, after enrolling in tutoring and cutting down my work hours, I retook the class and earned a better grade. I then went on to receive an A+ in a college-level calculus course.

Indicate the reasons for your specific interest in X University School of Medicine. (200 words or less)

    X is committed to nurturing talent and potential within its medical students to help them become leaders in medicine. This is evident through X's commitment to maintaining a diverse student body, and service to the diverse community of Y and beyond. Phenomenal faculty will allow me to learn the art of doctoring, and the scientific foundation necessary to be a great physician. Also, traditional scientific inquiry is an important part of scholarship. X has a strong neuroscience program which suits my research interests. X's educational philosophy of collaboration creates an environment in which I thrive. X's medical missions will allow me to contribute to the global community as I hope, through medicine, I will.

    The best medical school for me is one with which I share my core values. X is that school. I believe my diverse background and upbringing in the Y community will not only allow me to enhance the learning experience of my peers but the experiences of the patients I will serve. My commitment to lifelong learning, and desire to make a difference in the world illustrate my ability to uphold the values of X. I feel honored to be considered for a position.

List any particular medical specialties for your residency training in which you are interested. Your response does not affect admission and is used for statistical purposes only.

I hope to decide on a definitive path while in medical school. The following interests are a reflection of my experiences thus far:

- *Family Medicine*
- *Psychiatry*
- *Obstetrics and Gynecology*
- *Surgery*

Do you consider yourself a person who would contribute to the diversity of the student body of X University School of Medicine? (1000 characters or less)

I am a black man from San Francisco, with a passion for serving others. I have persevered through many challenges, some described elsewhere in my application. Unlike most other applicants, I chose to spend a fifth year in college; I completed medical school requirements, earned a bachelor's degree, explored personal interests (for example, became a certified personal trainer and served my community), and continued to hold a job to help support my family. I will have completed a year of full-time research at Z by the time I matriculate into medical school. All of these experiences have further cemented my decision to pursue medicine, and will undoubtedly allow me to practice better medicine. I hope to provide a unique perspective while collaborating with my prospective peers, and will be able to relate to a broader range of patients; I would be honored if given this opportunity.

Certain websites such as Student Doctor Network (SDN) allow you to access secondary essay questions other students post. Some students post actual secondary essay questions that they've accumulated throughout their admissions cycle. You can read these secondary essay prompts for more examples. See the Resource List. Just beware, there are some lunatics on SDN (don't take everything other students post as the final word). There are also a lot of negative students on SDN—remember, take everything with a grain of salt. Most of those students are not admissions experts.

If you complete enough secondaries, you will find that you can recycle essays from other secondaries you've completed. Medical schools often ask similar questions. It is okay to reuse an essay for a different secondary as long as it is your work. Just make sure you don't submit an essay to school X with school Y's name on it (this has happened)!

In summary, secondary applications may or may not add value to your candidacy for medical school. Some schools use them as an opportunity to learn more about you, others use them as a revenue stream. Either way, you don't want to be the one who takes the value away from your own application. Produce a good essay (doesn't have to be a masterpiece), be honest and positive, and PROOFREAD your essay! Remember to submit secondary applications promptly after you receive them to ensure you do not delay interview invitations.

12 INTERVIEWS

Okay, so you're almost across the finish line…almost. If you've made it this far and received an interview, your chances of being accepted to medical school are pretty high. The truth is that if you received an invitation to interview, most schools (not all) already believe that you can handle the academic rigor of medical school. Now they want to learn more about you and see if you're as good in person as you were on paper. This is not true for all schools as some medical schools interview a larger number of applicants (meaning they reject a larger proportion of them).

Early Preparation

Preparation for interviews has to begin long before you receive an interview invitation. There is one very important thing you can do from the moment you begin college: read the newspaper. I mentioned the importance of reading a reputable newspaper during the discussion about MCAT preparation. Not only will reading the paper help you with the verbal/critical reasoning section of the MCAT, but it will help prepare you for interviews.

Every applicant must be prepared to demonstrate that he or she is well-rounded and well-informed. This does not mean that you have to be an expert in politics, economics, foreign affairs and science. It just means that you need to be aware of what is going on in the world. The best thing to do is read the "front-page" of a newspaper's website. Read the headlines and first two paragraphs of each article. This will take you approximately 15 minutes per day.

There are some issues in which you must be well-versed for which you must read more than just the first few paragraphs. This may sound obvious but many students forget the importance of knowing about the healthcare system and medical education. Because you want to be a physician, you should know a fair amount about the American health care system and health care reform, as well as whether there are any major advancements in medical education. Again, you don't need to be an expert, spending hours reading about these issues. However, you should read articles related to these issues at a greater length or even read 1-2 books about these issues.

One easy tip I would highly recommend is to sign yourself up for Google Alerts. Google Alerts will use keywords you provide to search for articles on the internet and send the links to your email. With Google Alerts, you choose the topics and keywords. You can select "medical school," "health care reform," "health disparities," whatever you want! Then you select how frequently you want to receive your alerts (daily, weekly etc.). This way you can read stories from many different news sources all at once—you can even read blogs. It will probably feel overwhelming at first, but just reading the news for 30 minutes each day can have a cumulative effect that will prepare you to sound well-informed during interviews.

There are three questions you should think about long before your interview. You will be asked these exact three questions on almost every interview:

1. *Tell me about yourself.*
2. *Why do you want to be a physician?*
3. *Why do you want to attend our school?*

You already know all of the answers to the first question—you know yourself! However, you must choose the most important pieces of yourself to describe in order to make the right impression on your interviewer. A surprising amount of variation exists in the way in which people answer this question. Most interviewers will ask you this question to break the ice and make you feel more comfortable. However, this question often shows what your priorities are in life or what is important to you. For example, I always answer this question by talking about where I come from (New York City) and a bit about my family; I am multiracial and my parents divorced when I was young. My family life and New Yorker background directly contributed to my character and motivations for becoming a physician.

Don't feel obligated to speak about why you want to pursue medicine when you reply to "tell me about yourself." Talk about whatever you want. If you would like to do so, towards the end of your reply you can mention the reason why you want to become a physician. This allows for a natural transition to a new topic. The interviewer will either ask you to elaborate on something you said, or specifically to answer, "Why do you want to become a physician?"

After taking the time to reflect and write your personal statement and put together your application, you've probably thought about the following: why do you want to become a physician? Just make sure you can describe why you want to be a physician in less than three minutes. That's the tough part that requires practice. Come up with an "elevator pitch" to describe why you want to become a physician. Pretend you are trying to get your message across to an admissions committee member you meet in the elevator; before he gets off on his floor, you have to tell him why you want to be a physician. To give you a concrete example, in my answer to this question I mentioned my initial fascination with medicine as a child and then described the ways in which I explored the field throughout life. Finally, I summed it up by describing how I want to use medicine as a tool to enact change in the world. This answer was basically a much abbreviated version of what I wrote in my personal statement.

Finally, just as you read the paper to familiarize yourself with current events, you must familiarize yourself with the schools to which you are applying. In addition to reading about each school in the MSAR (previously discussed), visit each school's website. Read as much of it as you can—ideally, every section of the medical school's site and a bit about its affiliate hospitals. Find three things that make the school unique (e.g. pass/fail grading system, student-run health clinic, unique patient population etc.) and find two things you would like to learn more about (e.g. the culture of the school, the mentoring system etc.). By completing this exercise you are prepared to answer, "Why do you want to attend our school?" You are also prepared with two questions to ask at the end of the interview.

At the end of each interview, your interviewer will usually ask, "do you have any questions?" Some interviewers genuinely don't care if you take this opportunity to ask questions or not. Other interviewers will think you are disinterested if you don't have questions prepared. Since you will never know which type of interviewer you will have, make sure you prepare questions. Make sure the questions are thoughtful! If you can easily find the answer to your questions on the website, you are not only wasting your interviewer's time but will also appear to be careless.

In addition to preparing questions, whenever an interviewer asks whether you would like to add something—take advantage of this opportunity! Reiterate your interest in the school and why you are a good applicant (without bragging).

Once you finally have an invitation to interview, make sure that you reply right away. Do not wait to schedule your interview. Make sure that your emails are polite and courteous and use proper grammar, spelling, punctuation etc.

What to Wear

The other thing you can do fairly early in preparation for interviews is purchase your wardrobe. You want to project the right image when admissions committee members meet you for the first time. You need to look professional and well-kept. They should be able to envision you taking care of patients one day.

You will need at least two good suits. Not slacks and a blouse—suits. Think about fabric materials that will be good for the fall and winter as this is probably when you will interview. The best colors are black, gray and navy. These are the safest and most conservative colors. Trust me, you don't want to stand out for the wrong reasons on your interview day. You may also consider purchasing a third suit for warmer weather (depending on when and where you will interview). Your suits do not have to be expensive, just professional.

Women can wear either pants or a skirt with a matching jacket. Women should also wear a collared dress shirt underneath; white and blue shirts are the safest and most conservative. Stockings can be worn during colder weather should you decide to wear a skirt. Even in warmer weather, nude-colored stocking cannot hurt as this is the more conservative route. You should wear either flat or high-heeled dress shoes. Please keep in mind that you are not walking the catwalk in Paris—you don't need to look like a model or be the trendiest person on your interview day. You should feel like yourself and feel comfortable.

You can dress trendy if you'd like but only if the current trends are professional. You don't want to stand out. For example, around the time in which I interviewed, stilettos with a platform in the front became popular among the masses. If you don't know what I'm talking about, put lightly, these shoes look like exotic dancers' shoes. While this may be trendy and appropriate for dinner, clubs, weddings etc., it is never appropriate to wear these shoes on your interview day. Throughout all of my interviews I only saw one woman wearing such shoes, and she stuck out like a sore thumb. Like I said, you don't want to be remembered for the wrong reasons. Furthermore, make sure your shirts are not extremely low-cut, and your skirts fall just above your knee; miniskirts and cleavage are a no-no.

Also, a common component to almost every interview day is a campus tour. I highly recommend that you bring a second pair of super comfortable shoes to wear during the tour—maybe even throughout the entire day. These can be simple, flat shoes. You can always slip on your dressy shoes prior to going into your actual interview. On my first interview I did not do this, and my feet hurt for eight hours! I definitely remembered to bring comfortable shoes to my next interview.

Men should wear a simple suit. Solid is best. Thin pin-stripes are okay as long as the cut of the suit is appropriate. No pin-stripes in wild colors. Even a bowtie can seem like a gimmick (depending on how you wear it). Again, you do not want to be remembered for your appearance on your interview day.

Both men and women should cover tattoos, remove excessive or radical piercings. Women should either wear neutral colored nail polish, or no nail polish at all; if it is chipped, remove it before your interview. Men and women should not wear excessive jewelry and should wear a simple, natural hair style (no crazy colors, mohawks etc.).

Mock Interviews

How do you get to Carnegie Hall? Practice! The only way to get good at interviewing is to practice. It will help ease some of your anxiety. You can also receive constructive criticism from those who interview you and learn how to communicate, and to sound more natural and less nervous during the real thing.

Mock interviews are a must. You can do mock interviews as early as you would like in order to prepare for medical school interviews. Why not start sophomore year? You can ask professors, advisors and mentors to help you. You should also visit your school's professional development or career center to see if you can schedule a formal mock interview.

Stationery

Invest in blank stationery and stamps. You will have to send thank you notes after your interviews (more on this later) so it is worth buying a package of blank thank you cards from the drug store or convenience store. Do not spend a lot of money. Seriously, don't spend a lot of money. No one is going to judge you based on the cost of your stationery or the weight of the paper. You just need a basic set of stationery and stamps. Keep it professional (no comedic thank you cards, or immature cards that are pink with hearts and glitter). They *will* judge you if the stationery is unprofessional.

Know Your AMCAS

Become VERY familiar with your AMCAS application. You should know it inside and out, forwards and backwards. You should know the dates on which you began and ended an experience listed on your application. You should know your personal statement and every grade you got in every class. Be prepared to talk about anything and everything written in your application.

Interview Schedule and Format

Most interview days are similar. In the morning you meet for breakfast with other applicants. This is not true all the time so make sure you eat a complete breakfast at home. After breakfast there is usually an info session presented by the school; you may have an admissions person show you a PowerPoint presentation, interact with a panel of current students or even meet with the financial aid staff. You can have just one presentation or many. Then you have lunch and a campus tour. Throughout the day (sometimes all at once or each applicant at different times) you will have your interviews.

Most schools will give you one-on-one interviews with two different people. Some schools make you go through three interviews, some through one. These one-on-one interviews usually last 30 minutes to one hour. The person interviewing you may be a faculty member, physician, some other admissions person or even a medical student.

Take every interview seriously—even ones with medical students. No matter how relaxed the interviewer wants you to feel, always remember this is a medical school interview not a social event. Relax, but don't act unprofessionally. The other type of interview format gaining popularity is the multiple mini interview (MMI) format. While there is undoubtedly variation among medical schools, the MMI format goes something like this.

There are several different stations at which you will spend approximately five to ten minutes. An admissions committee member will be present at each station taking notes. The station may consist of a role playing game, presentation or discussion; you will not know which beforehand. This is supposed to make you think on your feet. For example, they may give you a clinical vignette about a patient and ask you to role play how you would convince the patient to quit smoking. Or the station may show you items to bring with you to medical school, but the catch is you can only bring three. They may ask you to choose three and explain why you chose them. MMI's are supposed to elicit other things about your personality that may not be readily apparent during a traditional interview. Whether or not this is true, is arguable but you should be aware of the format as you may encounter it. Here are a few other examples of MMI questions/stations:

> *With another student, debate whether marijuana should be legalized. You are pro-legalization.*

The key to answering this question is to be polite, professional and persuasive. Even if you don't know much about the issue, think of something thoughtful and try your best. This is a situation in which keeping up with current events will help you.

> *With three other students, build a free-standing structure using marshmallows and dried spaghetti.*

The goal here is not to build the tallest, strongest, structure. They just want to see how you interact with a team, share your ideas, direct others and listen. They want to make sure you are not overpowering, rude or a poor communicator.

> *You and a colleague are traveling to a professional conference. Your friend learns that her father has just passed away. Console her.*

THE HEARTBEAT OF SUCCESS

This station is testing your ability to think on your feet and demonstrate empathy and compassion. Even though this is not a real situation, do your best to console the other person. Don't go overboard and sound dramatic. You're not supposed to be acting, just trying to demonstrate what you would do in a similar, real situation.

A classmate tells you that he is falling behind in school. Help him.

This station seeks to demonstrate your ability to counsel others. Listen to your friend to gain knowledge, take the knowledge as well as knowledge you already have about school resources to help your friend come up with a game plan to improve his performance.

You are a medical student. The supervising resident mistreats a patient. What do you do?

This demonstrates how you handle conflict. You cannot be insubordinate but need to find a way start a dialogue with the resident. Be respectful at all times and try to listen to the resident's point of view.

Some schools participate in their own unorthodox practices. If you should find yourself in such a situation, don't worry—just be yourself. For example, one school asked me to write a 250-word essay about a photo they provided. They asked me to describe what was happening in the photo. The photo showed several different people waiting on a subway platform for the train to arrive.

I gave each person a story based on their outfits, describing from where each person came and where they were going. I even wrote a bit about what I thought the people were thinking based on their facial expressions. I'm sure if I had terrible writing skills this would have worked against me, but I think the real purpose of the essay was to elicit any underlying prejudices I may have had or to see how imaginative I am. Perhaps all they wanted to see was how I worked under pressure. Whatever the real reason, I made sure to do my best by following all of the aforementioned rules for writing essays and maintaining my professionalism.

Planes, Trains and Automobiles...and Couch Surfing

Many students often wonder how they will pay for or coordinate their interviews. The short answer: save money. Interviewing can be a very expensive process depending on where you interview and at how many schools. There are two things you can do to cut the costs of interviews.

Once your interview is scheduled, many schools will send you a list of current students who are willing to host you for the night before the big day. Take advantage of this opportunity! If you stay with a medical student host, you don't have to pay for lodging; even better, you get to pick the student's brain to learn about the school from a student's perspective. Often, medical students will be very honest. Just remember that when you stay with a medical student, you are still there for a medical school interview. You don't have to be fake, but don't complain if you have to sleep on the couch (although most students have an air mattress), don't brag about all the interviews or acceptances you have, don't drink, don't badmouth a school—in short, remain professional. Even though it is very unlikely, some medical students unofficially communicate with admissions staff sometimes (even if they say otherwise). Even if the student does not communicate with the admissions staff, make sure you are a good houseguest.

There is one more thing you can do to cut the cost of interviews. Let's say you live in California and a school in Chicago has invited you for an interview. You can contact the other schools in or near Chicago to which you applied, and let them know you will be in town for an interview. You do not have to disclose which school has invited you for an interview. Sometimes the other schools will make a decision about whether to interview you or not more quickly in order to accommodate you. Other times, they will tell you that they are not yet ready to make a decision in which case you have to suck it up and possibly fly to Chicago more than once.

This is a well-known and common practice that is permissible so don't be afraid to take advantage of it. As always, just make sure that your email is polite and professional. If you don't get the answer you want, politely thank the school and tell the staff you look forward to hearing from them in the future.

Finally, another thing you can do (that sometimes save you money) is partake in the usual travel saving-activities. Join mailing lists for discount airfare websites. You can set "fare alerts" on certain travel sites to receive notifications about low-price airfare. Join any special discount program or take advantage of student discounts various companies offer. Consider taking a bus or train instead of a plane (it is often cheaper). You may also want to work more to save money or ask family for help in order to pay for some expenses (if possible).

The Night Before

The night before your interview, give your AMCAS application one final read. Prepare your clothing for the next day (e.g. iron your suit). You also want to make sure that you have everything you need for the interview day (e.g. lip balm, lint brush, mints, hair gel etc.) What you decide to bring will be different from someone else—just bring whatever makes you comfortable. You should also have a pen with you, and something small to write on. In most instances, medical schools will give you promotional materials like pens and pads on the day you interview, but bring your own just in case they don't do so. If you have business cards, bring them. If you have a resume, bring a few copies (although this probably won't be necessary). Be sure to get a good night's rest! Be sure to get a good night's rest! Although you will undoubtedly be nervous, try to get a good night's rest. I cannot emphasize this enough. Interview days are long and you will undoubtedly be tired by the end so don't compound the problem by not sleeping enough.

The Day Has Finally Arrived

Your interview begins from the moment you step on campus. You never know whether or not the person standing next to you in the elevator will be the person interviewing you. Be courteous and polite to everyone you meet—even the security guard who gives you directions. Do not smoke cigarettes, drink alcohol or disclose personal business loudly on your cell phone. In fact, set your cell phone to silent. Do not play games on your phone, send text messages or read emails—admissions staff can misinterpret your behavior for disinterest. If you have to check your phone for any reason, go to the bathroom to do so.

Similar to your AMCAS application, electronic alter ego and wardrobe choice, you want to convey professionalism and maturity on your interview day. You want to be friendly, warm and demonstrate an interest in others. You can only do this if your cell phone is away, you are polite, and you make small talk with other applicants.

During one of my interview days, we were ready to begin the campus tour. I asked the medical student leading the tour whether I could quickly run to the bathroom to change my shoes. He said okay. When I returned from the bathroom three minutes later, the entire group had left! It was raining and I had no idea where to go. I decided to return to the admissions office and seek help. I explained what happened and after nearly 45 minutes, we found the tour group and I was able to rejoin. By the time I rejoined the group, the tour was ending and I had to run to the other side of campus for my first interview. What a mess.

Now between you and me, I was UPSET (and scared)! What type of medical student in charge of leading a tour group, leaves without making sure everyone is there? Even if he did not normally check attendance, I told him I was going to the bathroom. I know, I know—I realize that the medical student could have simply made a mistake. Nonetheless, when I returned to the admissions office for help, I was all smiles and sunshine. I tried to make light of the situation and emphasize how grateful I was for the admissions person's assistance (I really was grateful). I never let them know how upset I felt. You have to keep your cool and convey maturity and professionalism at all times.

I've sat in on several talks with admissions staff members from different medical schools. I've heard over and over again that "people are watching." I don't mean to make the admissions staff sound creepy but in a way they are! Remember that they are just looking for a reason to reject you. You are being watched at all times during your interview day, not just during your actual interview. Behave as you would in front of your future patients.

Make sure you make good eye contact throughout your actual interviews. Provide a firm, confident handshake at the beginning and end of your interview. Pause for a few seconds after each question so that you can think about your answer or at least look like you're thinking about your answer. You want to appear thoughtful and unrehearsed. It is tricky to strike a balance between practicing and appearing unrehearsed. This is why mock interviews are so important. Be aware of your body language as well. Sit tall with your hands on your lap or in some other relaxed position. Make sure you're not slouching or leaning on things, appearing too relaxed.

You need to sound like yourself and confident on your interview day. Do not brag but try to weave highlights from your application into your answers, where appropriate. Don't be afraid to say, "As you may have read in my application…" It is okay to repeat a lot of what is written in your application—it is your application after all. Do not sound too informal; you are not talking to your friend. This is your medical school interview.

At the end of the interview day, try to get your interviewers' contact information. This will probably have already been provided to you. If not, ask the admissions coordinator (do not ask your interviewer for his contact information). When you get home, write a hand-written thank you note on actual stationery (not loose leaf paper) and send the note to your interviewers. Some schools will specifically ask that you send electronic thank you notes via email. Others will simply say don't send thank you notes at all. Always follow the school's instructions. If they explicitly asked that you don't send a thank you note, and you send one, your disobedience could get you rejected. Also, if they say thank you notes are welcomed and you do not send one, you can appear ungrateful or unprofessional.

If you plan on sending a thank you note, do not wait more than 24 hours to send one. You can use almost the same message over and over for each note, just make sure you change the name and date where appropriate. Also, chances are that your thank you notes will be placed in your application file. Do not write two IDENTICAL notes. They can say the same thing (generally) but try to add at least one sentence that makes it personal. For example, "I really enjoyed learning more about the school and hearing how you decided to become a physician." Another note might have the same general message but the personal sentence may say, "I enjoyed meeting you and learning that you too cannot live without the subway system!"

Sample Interview Questions

I already spoke a bit about the questions for which you can prepare in advance. Aside from the aforementioned interview questions, I've listed some questions with advice about how to answer them. Please see the Resource List for more information.

If you were a part of a car, which part would you be and why?
I was asked this on one of my interviews. This question is not meant to be taken seriously. I think this question is silly, but the interviewer probably asked me this to see how I reacted under pressure. Additionally, my answer may have shed light on my personality. Was I the

headlights, guiding the car? The steering wheel, controlling the car? The radio, entertaining the driver? It doesn't really matter. The point is to take a breath, answer the question and just don't say anything crazy!

What are you passionate about?
Your answer does not have to be about medicine. Maybe you're simply passionate about being happy in life. Whatever you say, just be honest and again, don't say anything shocking or crazy. Don't say anything controversial. Keep it "G-rated." You can speak about your family, an extracurricular activity or hobby, exercise…whatever! If you're spiritual, don't be afraid to mention your spirituality- just make sure you don't degrade another religion.

What do you do to de-stress?
With this question, interviewers usually want to know two things: do you have a method for alleviating stress; is the method healthy? They want to make sure you have good coping skills, and that your coping skills are not self-destructive or harmful to others (e.g. no violence, cursing, screaming, alcohol or other drugs). Stress is unavoidable in medical school so they want to make sure you can find ways to manage stress.

Who do you rely on for support?
This question is similar to the last question except that it focuses more on external sources of support (rather than your coping skills alone). Your support system may

consist of friends, family, mentors or peers. Whatever you do, don't say you don't have a support system. Even if there is just one other person in the world you go to for help, mention that person.

What field of medicine do you want to pursue?
This is a tricky question. You need to demonstrate that you thought about your future but cannot come across as rigid or unrealistic. At this stage in your career, you probably have not had enough exposure to medicine to truly choose a field. Most medical students don't even know what field they like most. To safely answer this question, think about all of your experiences to date. If you have worked with children a lot, it's okay to say "I'm thinking about pediatrics right now, probably because I've worked with children so much. However, I have many interests and I'm keeping an open mind." Or you may say, "I am an athlete and underwent knee surgery. That experience got me interested in orthopedic surgery. Although I'd like to keep an open mind until I gain more clinical experience." Make sure you always say that you are keeping an open mind.

After the Interview

In addition to sending a thank you note, you need to debrief after each interview day. How did the interview go? What went well? What do you wish you would have done differently? Was there something that you did not explain well? Were you unfamiliar with a specific current event?

Just as with the MCAT, you need to review your interview behavior and performance. Do not harp on anything—this will only cause you stress. If you believe you need to improve on something, then get to work before your next interview. Do more mock interviews, read more about the healthcare system—do whatever you need to do to improve. Once you have pinpointed what should be improved, just focus on your next interview. As hard as it may be, don't replay your last interview in your head over and over (believe me I've been there).

The other thing you should do within 24 hours of completing your interview is to write 1-5 paragraphs about your impressions of the school. Describe the students, the vibe you felt, any good or bad gut feelings, interesting facts about the school or the surrounding neighborhood—whatever you want! Trust me, if you go on more than a few interviews everything will start to blur together. Therefore, it is very important to write your impressions of each school immediately following the interview. You will come back to these reflection pieces later.

13 ACCEPTANCES

And now, the moment you've all been waiting for...acceptances. But let's first talk logistics and a harsh reality.

Logistics

I'm sorry to be the bearer of bad news but the medical school application process is NOT as holistic as some medical schools and premedical advisors advertise. This was something I did not realize until I completed my own admissions cycle. Even then, I did not want to believe that the medical school application process is so political. However, after discussing my opinions with medical school administrators and other very reliable sources, I realize my opinions are facts.

During my interview cycle, while interviewing at a medical school in Chicago, I was repeatedly asked over and over whether I wanted to practice medicine in New York or not. I was asked about whether I was willing to leave New York for medical school. I was asked how many schools I applied to outside the state of New York. At the time, I was just honestly answering the questions and could not understand why everyone cared so much about how much I love New York.

It turns out that the admissions staff members were gauging my interest in their school and trying to gauge my willingness to leave New York and actually move to Chicago. Why would they care about this so much? They were afraid I would reject them. That's right. As badly as you want to avoid rejection, medical schools want to avoid rejection too. When they accept an applicant and then an applicant chooses another school it messes up their statistics; if many accepted applicants end up turning the school down, it can make the school (on paper) look undesirable. The more students apply to a school, and the less the school accepts, the more exclusive the school looks. It looks even better when all of the accepted applicants choose to go to that school—hello, prestige! Therefore, it came as no surprise to me that I was waitlisted at the Chicago school despite a great interview day.

Whether they admit it or not, medical schools care very deeply about statistics. Statistics allow one school to be compared to another (even if the statistics they use are meaningless in real life). For each new incoming class each year, medical schools usually come up with a statistical profile for the students: how many students are state residents, male or female, underrepresented minority (also known as diversity), the average undergraduate

GPA, the average MCAT score, and how many universities are represented within the incoming class.

The reason why the MCAT and your undergraduate GPA are so important is because your "metrics" can either bring down or bring up a school's statistics. Medical schools prefer to admit applicants that improve or have no effect on their numerical profile. If you are going to bring down a school's statistics, they will only accept you if extenuating circumstances affected your "metrics" or they need a student like you to improve their profile (e.g. you are disadvantaged, they want to increase diversity and you are a minority in some way, you have a wonderfully unique story that describes your interest in medicine etc.). For example, you may be rejected because they really needed another out-of-state resident in the incoming class versus an in-state resident, or because they need a Hispanic male instead of a Hispanic female.

Therefore, whether or not you are accepted to medical school has a lot to do with circumstances that are out of your control. It is for this reason that you will hear many use the word "crapshoot" to describe the medical school admissions process. I wouldn't call it a crapshoot entirely. You do have a fair amount of control over your application. If you do everything right, use the guidance provided in this book, medical schools won't want to reject you—they will want to offer you admission. Keep in mind that there will always be a few (sometimes more than a few) who may choose to reject you because they think you will turn them down, or you will bring down their statistics and thus their prestige.

This is something many premedical advisors, admissions representatives and physicians won't tell you. This is not something they will say on the record. Off the record, many (if not all) will confirm what I have said. I feel it is absolutely essential that I be forthcoming with you about this harsh reality because as I mentioned, this was something I learned only after completing the admissions process. Prior to applying to medical school, I held the admissions process on a pedestal.

Had I learned a bit earlier about the way in which admissions really works, I would have taken rejection a little bit more in stride. I don't want you to get too down on yourself, should you not be accepted to medical school the first time around, or not be accepted to your top-choice medical school. The sooner you know the way the medical school application process works, the more you can ponder and come to terms with it.

The Good Stuff

Most schools participate in rolling admissions, as described earlier. Therefore, you will know whether or not you've been accepted to medical school during the several weeks following your interview. There are some exceptions to this rule (e.g. the first round of acceptances are released after a certain date, all acceptances are released on the same day etc.). The best place to search for the most up-to-date information is on the school's website or in the MSAR.

If you are accepted to a medical school....YAY! CELEBRATE! Congratulations! You did it. You succeeded at one of the most difficult screening processes on the road to becoming a physician. For every school that accepts you, you must submit a deposit to hold your place in the class. Your deposit will be refunded if you choose not to attend a school and make the decision before a certain date (each school can specify its own date but it is usually during the second week of May preceding the start of the school year). It is important to hold a place in every school to which you are accepted because you can later use these acceptances as bargaining chips.

Let's say you are accepted to schools X, Y and Z. X offered you a 50% merit-based tuition scholarship for all four years of medical school. Y offered you a 75% merit-based tuition scholarship for all four years, but Z only offered you a 20% merit-based tuition scholarship for all four years. The school you REALLY want to go to is Z. You can politely approach the admissions staff at Z via email and let them know that you received a 75% scholarship from another school and ask if they are able to match it. You don't have to tell them at which schools you were accepted, although after a certain date AMCAS releases this information to every school anyway. The admissions committee will then discuss whether they want to give you a larger scholarship at their next admissions meeting.

Trust me, EVERYONE who has more than one acceptance participates in this practice. Take advantage of it. Medical schools are used to receiving these types of requests and the worst thing that can happen is a school will simply tell you "no." I was very afraid to ask medical schools for more money as the practice seemed so unorthodox to me. However, my mentors advised me properly; I'm glad I was pushed to be a bit more assertive.

The one thing I regret is that I withdrew my application from consideration from a handful of schools. I was invited for so many interviews and quickly running out of money so I had to withdraw my application before I even interviewed. In hindsight this was a mistake because those interviews could have led to even more acceptances and thus bargaining chips. If you have the money to go on all the interviews you receive, do it! It will be worth it should you receive more acceptances.

If you receive more than one acceptance, you will perhaps have to make the hardest (but best) decision of your life—you will have to choose a medical school. The scholarship issue I mentioned earlier might be the only thing that influences your decision. Many students choose to go to the medical school that offers them the best scholarship and financial aid package in an effort to save money. This is a perfectly good way to choose a school, but there are other factors you may consider.

As with everything else, you should do what you love and go to the school you liked the best. Throughout my interviews, most of the current medical students described that they experienced a "gut feeling" during their interview at a particular school, which later made them decide to attend that school. I must admit, I also felt that "gut feeling" at my medical school. However, not everyone will feel this, and that was not the only thing that influenced my decision.

Other medical students I met had very logical reasons for choosing the school they chose. For example, it was their state school and thus cheaper or closer to home, they were accepted to a special degree program at the school (e.g. MD/PhD, MD/MPH etc.), the school had a unique patient population, they wanted to work with a specific faculty member at the school, the grading system is pass/fail, the students were very friendly etc. Regardless of which school of thought you follow regarding choosing a medical school, you have to make sure you will be happy with your decision.

Review your post-interview reflection pieces. If you really want to get logical, you can translate all of your qualitative observations into quantitative data. You can come up with a scoring rubric and give each school one point for meeting a criterion on your rubric. Then you can add up the total points for each school and choose the school with the highest number of points, or at least narrow down your list using this method.

I would like to share with you what I think is most important about a medical school. The truth is that you will learn the same thing at every school you attend. You will take the same licensing exam and become a doctor no matter where you attend medical school. What makes the difference, is the environment in which you will learn. For me, a pass/fail grading system during the first two years of medical school was and still is absolutely non-negotiable. I cannot even imagine how students survive a traditional grading system during the first two years. I tip my hat to them. With the pass/fail system, my classmates and I still study harder than ever but we are more collaborative. We also feel okay cutting back on the studying in order to pursue extracurricular activities. This keeps us sane and balanced.

The other thing that helps ease the competitiveness of medical school is the absence of an internal ranking system. Some schools say they're pass/fail during the first two years, and they are; but they also use students' test grades to rank each student compared to her peers. So the transcript grade is pass/fail but the actual test grades you earn do contribute to your class ranking. I would explicitly ask about this during interviews and avoid schools that do this. Who needs the extra stress?

Also, I don't care how smart you are or how mature and diligent you are, you will definitely experience challenges in medical school. What determines how well you overcome these challenges is a) how supportive the administration is and b) how supportive your prospective classmates will be. During interviews, you should ask the current medical students (NOT your interviewer): what happens if you fail an exam? If you fail a class? If you fail the year? Is the environment collaborative or competitive? What do the medical students do for fun? What is the mentoring system (formal or informal) like at the school? The answers to these questions can give you an idea of what the culture is like at the school. When the going gets tough, you want to make sure you can lean on your peers for support and can rely on the administration to do everything in its power to help you.

The last thing I think really matters about a medical school is whether or not you have contact with patients during the first two years of school. Having completed my first year of medical school I can tell you that no matter how hard the school tries to make basic science material clinically relevant, it is still basic science material. At times it will drive you nuts, especially if you decided to go to medical school to work with and help people. Therefore, early patient contact can really motivate you and remind you about the reasons you decided to become a physician in the first place. Even if you only work with patients once per month that is sometimes all you need to stay motivated. Patient contact can occur via the formal curriculum, extracurricular activities or working for the student-run clinic.

Rejection

So you didn't get in. Now what. First of all, breathe. I promise you it is not the end of the world although it may feel that way. Think about this book's earlier discussions about choosing to retake a class you failed or choosing to retake the MCAT. You can only reapply to medical school once you've done two things.

The first thing you must do is analyze why you may have been rejected. Unfortunately, medical schools will not provide you with any feedback. Therefore, it is essential that you find a mentor who is encouraging but also honest. This mentor should have some sort of medical school admissions experience. You need to work with your mentor to figure out weaknesses within your application. Do you need a better MCAT score? Do you need to revise your personal statement? Do you need to improve your interview skills?

Sometimes, the things that most worked against you during the admissions cycle, you cannot change. For example, if you've already completed undergraduate school, you cannot change your academic record or GPA. If something like this is truly what had a negative impact on your medical school application there are several things you can consider doing.

You might consider taking graduate level science courses and working your hardest to do well. If you do well in these graduate courses, it will prove to medical school that not only are your days of poor grades behind you, but that you are prepared to handle graduate level science courses like those in medical school. You can also consider joining a post-baccalaureate program designed specifically for second-time applicants to medical school.

These post-baccalaureate programs do not offer a degree and instead offer one of all of the following: advanced science coursework; remedial science coursework; MCAT preparation; interview preparation; guaranteed acceptance to medical school. That's right, guaranteed acceptance to medical school. For example, let's say that you join a post-baccalaureate program for second-time applicants at University X. University X may have certain criteria, which if you meet them, you will automatically be accepted to University X's medical school the next year. Depending on the school, criteria may include retaking the MCAT and getting a certain minimum score, taking science classes within the medical school and earning a certain minimum GPA. Please visit the Resource List for more information about some of these programs.

If your weakness was not academic, figure out what it was and work to improve it. I know of one true story in which a man was rejected from medical school. After meeting with his mentor he determined his personal statement needed to be revised. The following admissions cycle he submitted the same exact application with one difference: an improved essay. The man was then accepted to more than one medical school! Once you have determined what went wrong, you may need to spend a year engaging in more clinical experiences, spend time revising your personal statement, schedule more mock interviews, retake the MCAT or find a research project; you may even need to do a combination of more than one of these things. Again, the solution is different for every individual.

One of the most important personal attributes in life is the ability to persevere and overcome adversity. It is important to face your challenges head on and learn from each bump in the road. This is something medical schools also admire as the ability to persevere is essential to be a successful medical student and eventually, a good physician. Everyone experiences hardship at one point or another during medical training. Continue to pursue your passions, and don't be afraid to apply to medical school again.

14 THE SUMMER BEFORE MED SCHOOL

So…you've been accepted and chose a school. What should you do to prepare for medical school? The answer is simple…as little as possible! I don't mean you should drop out of school, quit your job and become a recluse. I simply mean don't do ANYTHING to prepare for medical school. You're already prepared.

You should spend your time before beginning medical school enjoying yourself. You have no idea how lucky you are to have immense amounts of free time (relative to that of a medical student). If you would like to travel, travel. If you would like to work to save money, work. If you would like watch the entire series of Scrubs on Netflix, go for it (this is what I did)! You should also consider spending time with friends and family. While you're not going off to war, once school begins you will be studying A LOT. Take advantage of your guilt-free free time while you have it.

One important activity you should do is think about how you learn best. I cannot emphasize this enough. The truth is you might not know exactly how you study best until you get to medical school. However, the sooner you begin to think about what type of learner you are and what type of study methods work best for you, the better. In addition to challenging your ability to manage your time, medical school challenges you as a learner as well. Please see the Resource List for some websites that address this topic.

Finally, you should leave some room for celebration. If you are preparing to begin medical school, you've gotten through one of the hardest parts of becoming a physician. While there are many challenges ahead, it's okay to feel relieved for a bit and pat yourself on the back. Engage in self-reflection and think about what is important to you in life. Write down your values on a piece of paper. I promise you that medical school will challenge your beliefs in many ways. It's very easy to forget why you wanted to become a physician in the first place when you are busy studying basic science coursework, and to consider fields of medicine like dermatology simply because you saw your tuition bill—don't let this happen to you.

Any time you feel lost, pull out your piece of paper and read about all of things that helped you reach this point in your life. Don't ever forget who you are, where you come from or where you are going.

15 STORIES FOR INSPIRATION

PC lived on a farm in Colombia with his parents and four siblings. Agricultural conditions were terrible; they were starving and indigent. His mother immigrated to the Bronx where she lived by herself in an abandoned building to avoid paying rent. She got a job in construction doing manual labor working 40 to 60 hours per week and babysat most of the rest of the time.

Meanwhile, PC was in Colombia being schooled in a one room school house. He had to walk 1 ½ miles to school without shoes – he could not afford them. He did not possess any books; they were all in school. Finally, PC's mother saved enough to get the rest of the family to the Bronx, where they now could afford to rent an apartment. His father left and his mother had to raise all five children on her own. PC was 13 years old at the time.

PC's family taught him that education was the answer to everything. PC attended high school in New York City (one of the city's worst high schools). He could not afford any formal English courses and learned English on his own. Despite this, he was still able to graduate as valedictorian of his high school class. He heard that attending a top university would improve his chances of becoming a physician and was accepted to an Ivy League school; he received no scholarship support – only loans. PC graduated from Ivy League University with a 2.5 GPA. His total MCAT score was 20. He was then rejected by 20 medical schools.

He retook the MCAT and got a 22 while he worked as a Research Associate, taught in an underserved area of New York City and volunteered in a health clinic. Meanwhile, he earned a master's degree in science from a prestigious university with a 3.8 GPA. His third MCAT score was 24 and he was accepted to medical school in New York City in 2007.

During all of his free time in medical school, he worked with poor immigrants in the Bronx, teaching them health literacy and preventive medicine. He continued to work in the health clinic. He ultimately received an award of recognition from the city.

He successfully graduated from medical school. He aced Steps 1 and 2 of the United States Medical Licensing Exam (USMLE), volunteered as a teaching assistant for Anatomy, and is on his way to be a family medicine doctor in the Bronx. He matched to his top-choice residency program. At graduation, he received two prestigious awards. As a side note, all of PC's siblings graduated from college; one just earned his PhD. To this day, their mother can neither read nor write Spanish or English.

AB was born in New York City. Both parents were drug addicts and in prison for a large part of AB's life. At an early age AB became a ward of the state. She bounced from foster home to foster home and realized as a teenager that she could be a doctor. During high school, she supported herself with a full time factory job. AB then went to a public university and earned a 3.0 GPA. She joined a mentoring organization as she was finishing college. Her MCAT score was a 25.

AB is now a third year medical student at a Midwestern medical school with a 100% scholarship! She did well during her first semester. Her score on Step 1 of the USMLE was higher than her school's average and higher than the national average. AB is well on her way to becoming a fantastic physician!

AB (from the previous story) had a friend named DP, and they always studied together. DP lived in poor area of New York City and also had to work while going to college. DP's motivation for pursuing medicine stemmed from a long hospitalization she experienced after being in a motor vehicle accident. Like AB, she went to a public university and earned a 3.0 average. Her MCAT score was 23 (VR7, PS7, BS9). She was accepted to and is doing well in a historically black medical school in the Southern United States.

X applied to 21 schools with 21 rejections. He went to Duke University as an undergraduate. His science GPA was 2.7 and overall 3.26. His MCAT score was 25. He got a D in organic chemistry, C- in biochemistry, C- in physics, W in two biology courses, another C in physics, and 3 other C's in two chemistry courses and a biology course. His essay was terrible; he devoted a lot of time to his fear of animal research and how he didn't like research. He reapplied to 13 schools with a new essay, repeated organic chemistry and earned an A-, did some research, more community service, honed his interview skills and was accepted to three medical schools.

Y graduated from Johns Hopkins University with a 2.7 GPA in science and a 3.1 overall GPA. This included an F in Organic Chemistry I, F in Organic Chemistry II, C and C- in Physics I and II, respectively. She also received a C in Calculus. Her MCAT score was 21 (BS7, PS7, VR7). She did not apply then but instead got her master's degree in public health with 6 Passes, 5 B's, 6 A's. She retook biochemistry and earned a C and unfortunately failed Organic Chemistry a second time. She retook the MCAT and earned a 25 (BS9, PS9, VR7). She was interviewed by eight schools and accepted to three in total. She received a full scholarship from one school, where she is currently doing well.

LMO came here from Sierra Leone in June 2006, knowing no English (spoke French and an African dialect), and lived in an underserved area of New York

THE HEARTBEAT OF SUCCESS

City. She lived with her mother who knows minimal English and lost her job because of significant illness. She was told that medical school was an impossible dream. She attended a public university as a pre-nursing student.

For a year before college, she worked while learning English. She earned a perfect 4.0 GPA in 92 credits of biology, chemistry, physics and math, and 3.99 total GPA. Her MCAT score was a 26 (BS10, PS10, VR6). She also did a lot of community service.

LMO was so disappointed in her MCAT that she wanted to delay her applications and apply the following year. She ultimately submitted her application and an Ivy League school invited her for an interview. She received nine acceptances including an acceptance to Ivy League University. Ivy League University gave her a full 4-year tuition scholarship plus additional spending money. During medical school, she also won a $100,000 scholarship.

QT went to college in upstate New York. She became interested in medicine after she received great care during a medical crisis of her own. Another unique aspect of her application was that she was over the age of 30. QT earned a D- in general chemistry, C in Chemical Analysis, C in math, C+ in biology, C+ in genetics, 2 more C's in biology courses. Her overall GPA was 3.0. The first time she took the MCAT she scored a 20 (BS5, PS6, VR9). She was told to forget about medicine.

For the next few years QT did research and was a lab technician. She retook the MCAT four years later and scored a 17 (BS5, PS4, VR8). She spent a few years completing post-baccalaureate courses at a large public university. Her grades included 18 As, 2 Bs and 1 C. During this time she also worked at least three jobs, and cared for an ill family member. Her third MCAT score was a 26 (BS9, PS8, VR9). She applied to eighteen schools, received twelve interviews and four acceptances.

CJ came from Trinidad and Tobago and is 35 years old. He went to Morehouse College and majored in economics and was a successful management consultant in several leadership positions for six years. He also spent significant time volunteering with the disabled and underserved. With the economy taking a turn for the worst and seeing the benefits of a medical doctorate, he completed a post-baccalaureate program. He earned two years of straight As and Bs. His MCAT score was a 25 (BS8, PS9, VR8). He was successfully accepted to medical school.

OJ was rejected from medical school with an undergraduate GPA of 3.77 from a large, public university. His MCAT was less than 20. He reapplied after retaking the MCAT and scored a 23 (BS8, PS9, VS6). He was accepted to a school in the Caribbean as well as one school in New York City.

PBJ immigrated to the United States as an adolescent. He worked full-time throughout college. He graduated from a large, public university with a 3.32

average, as a biochemistry major. He was devastated when his MCAT score was an 18. He retook it and earned a 23. He took the MCAT a third time and earned a 28. He had several interviews and was accepted to five medical schools.

JP graduated from Wesleyan. Her science GPA was 2.73 and overall GPA was 2.99, which included 3 Ds in three chemistry courses and a C- in Organic Chemistry. She also received a C- in biology. Over the next two years she completed a post-baccalaureate program at a large, public school and earned a 3.36 GPA; she took one or two courses per semester (most of the courses were repeats). Her first MCAT score was 22 (BS8, VR6, PS8). She also did significant work for the poor and underserved.

One year later, JP's second MCAT score was 26 (BS9, VR8, PS9). She was rejected by all 27 schools to which she applied. However, she was accepted to several post-baccalaureate programs to better prepare her for medical school. After completing a post-baccalaureate program, she was accepted to a large, state medical school where she is now a second year medical student and breezing through the coursework. She passed Step 1of the USMLE with flying colors.

LL graduated from a large, public university in New York City. She majored in biology. She was also a varsity athlete. She did not consider herself disadvantaged even though her father was disabled because there was always food on the table, unlike many of her friends. She lived in a dangerous neighborhood in New York City, and Spanish was the only language spoken at home.

LL did not apply to medical school until two years after graduating from college, primarily because of her low MCAT score of 23 (BS9, PS8, VR6). By contrast, her undergraduate GPA was practically all As with a handful of Bs (2.5 overall GPA). She retook the MCAT and earned a 25 (BS8, PS10, VR7), and completed a post-baccalaureate program, earning mostly Bs. She was finally accepted to five medical schools.

ST graduated from NYU with a 2.86 overall GPA. She received a full scholarship and had to work part time during her college career. She also did a lot of volunteer work with patients. A few months after graduation, her MCAT results were 28 (BS10, PS10, VR8). After graduation, she did research and despite several interviews, she received no acceptances. She completed a post-baccalaureate program at a large university in her home state. She earned straight As and Bs. She was successfully admitted to one medical school in New York City.

PV grew up in Pennsylvania and received a four-year scholarship to Swarthmore where she majored in religious studies and had a 3.6 GPA. Spanish was her primary language until college. All her premed requirements were taken as a post-baccalaureate student since she did not take any science classes as an undergraduate; she earned straight As. Her first MCAT score was 21 (BS9, PS9, VR3). She retook the exam and earned a 25 (BS9, PS11, VR5). She received two acceptances to medical school.

JD came from Nigeria at the age of nine and lived with a large extended family in New York City. Money had to be sent back to Nigeria to help support many other close relatives. He had to work from an early age but achieved an overall GPA of 3.7 from a large, public university which included a B in Biochemistry, A in Genetics, B in Molecular Biology, and an A in Physical Chemistry. He tutored, did research and was involved in church activities. His first MCAT score was 17 (BS5, PS9, VR3); second MCAT score was 19 (BS8, PS7, VR4); his third MCAT score (three weeks later) was 23 (BS8, PS7, VR8). He was accepted to two medical schools.

XI had to work 15-20 hours per week while she attended college and graduated with a 3.2 overall GPA (she earned a C+ in Organic Chemistry). She received a master's degree in public health from Ivy League University, earning fourteen As and two Bs. Additionally, she devoted a tremendous time to not only caring for the poor but working on public policy. She devoted herself to health disparities in the USA for five years and then decided it was time to apply to medical school. She was devastated when she received her MCAT score: 23. However, she was called for several interviews and was accepted to three medical schools.

RO graduated from a large, public university with an overall GPA of 3.52 and a 3.41 science GPA. His MCAT score was 29 (BS10, PS11, VR8). He received three interviews and was rejected by the twelve schools to which he applied. After he received his master's degree, he reapplied to ten schools, received three interviews and ten rejections. He then joined a mentoring program, partook in community service activities and retook the MCAT earning a 30 (BS12, PS10, VR8). He also practiced his interpersonal and interview skills and applied to a total of 35 medical schools. He received ten interviews and three acceptances.

ACKNOWLEDGEMENTS

I would like to express my deepest gratitude to my mentors, Dr. Irwin Dannis and Dr. Lynne Holden, without whom this book would not be possible: their wisdom and encouragement allowed me to be a successful medical school applicant and inspired me to write this book. I can only hope to influence someone else's life the way they have influenced mine. I would like to thank Andrew Morrison and Small Business Camp for sponsoring the book writing challenge that provided me the motivational fuel to push my book across the finish line. Many thanks to Dr. Ann-Gel Palermo, Dr. Gary Butts and the CMCA family for their unwavering support. Finally, I would like to thank Jennifer Betancourt, Frank Wolf, the Jeannette K. Watson Fellowship, Mentoring in Medicine, Inc., Debra Kennedy, the CCNY SEEK Program, and Dr. Jennifer Walden for taking me under their wings and preparing me for my journey in the field of medicine.

RESOURCE LIST

Association of American Medical Colleges (AAMC)
https://www.aamc.org/

American Medical College Application Service (AMCAS)
https://www.aamc.org/students/applying/amcas/

Career Exploration Websites
- Aspiring Docs:
  https://www.aamc.org/students/aspiring/
- Explore Health Careers:
  http://explorehealthcareers.org/en/home
- Health and Human Services Poverty Guidelines, 2011
  http://aspe.hhs.gov/poverty/11poverty.shtml

Interviews
- Kansagra, Sujay. Why Medicine? And 500 Other Questions for the Medical School and Residency

Interview. CreateSpace Independent Publishing Platform. 2012. Print.

- Interview Skills Consulting Medical School Interview Questions: http://www.medical-interviews.co.uk/interview-questions-medical-school-interviews.aspx

Learning Style/Study Methods

- Dartmouth Academic Skills Center: Improving Concentration, Memory, and Motivation http://www.dartmouth.edu/~acskills/success/study.html
- Lawrence, Gordon D. Looking at Type and Learning Styles: Using Psychological Type to Make Learning Personally Effective. 4th ed. Gainesville: Center for Applications of Psychological Type, Inc., 2007. Print.
- UC San Diego School of Medicine Educational Support Services: http://meded.ucsd.edu/index.cfm//ugme/oess/study_skills_and_exam_strategies//how_to_study_actively/

- University of South Dakota: What's YOUR Learning Style?
  http://sunburst.usd.edu/~bwjames/tut/learning-style/

MCAT

- AAMC's 2013 MCAT Essentials:
  https://www.aamc.org/students/download/63060/data/mcatessentials.pdf
- AAMC's Information about the 2015 MCAT:
  https://www.aamc.org/students/applying/mcat/mcat2015/
- AAMC Practice MCATs:
  https://www.aamc.org/students/applying/mcat/preparing/85158/orderingpracticetests_mcat.html
- Fee Assistance Program (FAP):
  https://www.aamc.org/students/applying/fap/
- Medical Minority Applicant Registry (Med-MAR):
  https://www.aamc.org/students/minorities/med-mar/

Mentoring in Medicine, Inc.:
http://www.medicalmentor.org

Personal Statement
- The Staff of The Princeton Review. Medical School Essays That Made a Difference. 4th ed. New York: Random House, Inc., 2012. Print.

Professional Organizations
- American Medical Student Association: http://www.amsa.org/AMSA/Homepage/MemberCenter/Premeds.aspx
- American Medical Women's Association: http://www.amwa-doc.org/
- Latino Medical Student Association: http://lmsa.net/
- Student National Medical Association: http://www.snma.org/premedical.php

Student Doctor Network: http://studentdoctor.net/

Summer Opportunities

- AAMC Program Search:
  http://services.aamc.org/summerprograms/
- Columbia University's List of Summer Biology Internships:
  http://www.columbia.edu/cu/biology/ug/intern.html
- Jeannette K. Watson Fellowship:
  http://www.jkwatson.org/
- Mentoring in Medicine, Inc.:
  http://www.medicalmentor.org/about/team.html
- Summer Medical and Dental Education Program:
  http://www.smdep.org/apply.htm
- Summer Undergraduate Research Programs:
  https://www.aamc.org/members/great/61052/great_summerlinks.html
- Ventures Scholars Program's List of Enrichment Programs for High School Students:
  http://www.venturescholar.org/hs/enrichment.htm

National Institutes of Health Programs

- Summer Internship Program in Biomedical Research:
  https://www.training.nih.gov/programs/sip
- NIH Academy:
  https://www.training.nih.gov/new_nih_academy_home
- Post-Baccalaureate Intramural Research Training Award:
  https://www.training.nih.gov/programs/postbac_irta
- Technical Intramural Research Training Award:
  https://www.training.nih.gov/programs/tech_irta
- Undergraduate Scholarship Program:
  https://www.training.nih.gov/programs/ugsp

Scholarships and Fellowships

- Barry Goldwater Scholarship:
  http://www.act.org/goldwater/#
- Boren Award:
  http://www.borenawards.org/boren_scholarship

- Fulbright Award:
  http://www.fulbrightteacherexchange.org/
- Harry S. Truman Scholarship:
  http://www.truman.gov/
- Marshall Scholarship:
  http://www.marshallscholarship.org/
- Mellon Mays Undergraduate Fellowship:
  http://www.mmuf.org/
- National Science Foundation Scholarships:
  https://www.nsf.gov/funding/pgm_summ.jsp?pims_id=5257
- Rhodes Scholarship:
  http://www.rhodesscholar.org/
- Soros Fellowships for New Americans:
  http://www.pdsoros.org/
- Thomas J. Watson Fellowship:
  http://www.watsonfellowship.org/site/index.html

ABOUT THE AUTHOR

Alexa M. Mieses is a second-year medical student at the Icahn School of Medicine at Mount Sinai in New York City. She is pursuing an MD/MPH joint-degree, and aspires to work with underserved populations as a primary care physician. A native New Yorker, Ms. Mieses graduated from the prestigious Bronx High School of Science before earning a B.S. in biology from the City University of New York. She attributes her success to wonderful mentorship and is passionate about mentoring others.

Made in the USA
Middletown, DE
15 December 2016